Sun & Ssukgat

The Korean Art of Self-Care, Wellness & Longevity

Michelle Jungmin Bang

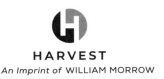

HARVEST
An Imprint of WILLIAM MORROW

HarperCollins books may be purchased for educational, business, or sales promotional use. For information, please email the Special Markets Department at SPsales@harpercollins.com.

FIRST EDITION

Designed by Melissa Lotfy and Hampton Agency
Photographs and illustrations by Michelle Jungmin Bang
Photograph on page 77 © CameraBalboa/Shutterstock

Library of Congress Cataloging-in-Publication Data
Names: Bang, Michelle Jungmin, author.
Title: Sun & ssukgat : the Korean art of self-care, wellness & longevity /
    Michelle Jungmin Bang.
Other titles: Sun and ssukgat
Description: First edition. | New York, NY : Harvest, an imprint of William
    Morrow, [2025] | Includes index. |
Identifiers: LCCN 2024033671 (print) | LCCN 2024033672 (ebook) | ISBN
    9780063341524 (hardcover) | ISBN 9780063436664 | ISBN 9780063436671 |
    ISBN 9780063341531 (ebook)
Subjects: LCSH: Self-help techniques. | Self-help techniques—Korea. |
    Longevity. | Longevity—Korea. | Self-care, Health. | Well-being.
Classification: LCC BF632 .B26 2025 (print) | LCC BF632 (ebook) | DDC
    613.09519—dc23/eng/20241104
LC record available at https://lccn.loc.gov/2024033671
LC ebook record available at https://lccn.loc.gov/2024033672

ISBN 978-0-06-334152-4

25 26 27 28 29 VPI 10 9 8 7 6 5 4 3 2 1

For my family

Contents

Ssukgat

The power of ssukgat, the gold-crested garland chrysanthemum, can easily go unnoticed. But this plant is more than an ornamental flower. Its healing abilities have been treasured and passed down for centuries in Korea. To find ssukgat today, you have to search by one of its multitude of names—Chinese Tong Ho, Japanese Shungiku, or crown daisy. To grow it, you can plant its seeds; or you can coax one of its withered stalks to bloom again with soil, sun, water, and care. Thus, ssukgat can be rekindled many times over, growing new roots each time as if reborn.

Introduction

Self-care

The practice of actively protecting one's health and well-being.

Self-care is the radical and yet centuries-old notion of taking a proactive rather than a reactive approach to wellness. It means focusing on the little things you can do every day to feel better, and in so doing, living a longer and more vibrant life by avoiding preventable illness and premature aging. This is simple wisdom that my ancestors practiced long ago—wisdom that should be preserved and not forgotten.

In Korean culture, food means love and self-care

In Korean families, love and concern are veiled rather unexpectedly in food expressions. "Have you eaten yet?" is really code for "How are you?" Go deeper still, and it means: "Are you taking good care of yourself?" These nuanced translations tie back to long-held beliefs in Korean traditions, where food is inextricably tied to love and self-care. **In Korea, food means more than filling our bellies; it means comfort, community, and our first medicine,** which we use to nourish and to let the body heal.

For centuries, Koreans have used simple cures like home-cooked meals with specific ingredients to treat ailments and prevent early symptoms from becoming chronic, or perhaps even irreversible. My family fed me these dishes as a child whenever I fell ill. These were nourishing recipes from our Korean culture, brought across the ocean to Brooklyn, where I was born and raised by my immigrant parents. When I had the stomach flu, my mother used to make juk, a warm and comforting rice porridge, easily digestible and ideal for the sick. In the summer, my father cooked samgyetang, a soup made with chicken stuffed with ginseng and glutinous rice. It's packed with nutrients to replenish those lost from sweating during the hottest days. And my grandmother made my favorite doenjang jjigae, a fermented bean stew, full of gut-healthy probiotics, protein-rich tofu, and melty zucchini. This nourishing welcome-home meal during my visits back from college filled me with joy; I knew she made this for me because she remembered that I loved this dish best.

As I grew older and moved away from my Brooklyn home, eventually settling in both Hong Kong and Manhattan, I often thought about my family's healing recipes from childhood. As a burnt-out entrepreneur, I had strayed far from the Korean wisdom of taking good care of myself. Like so many of us, I realized that the stresses and lifestyle choices of modern life were not only destroying my body and my peace of mind but also harming the planet.

One morning, while walking along Hong Kong's Stanley Beach and noodling on this, I saw a group of seniors in bathing suits gathering. Catching a glimpse of their energy and supple skin, these silvered elders looked more like young athletes from a distance. They had coordinated an outdoor activity together, alternating between doing vigorous laps in the ocean and deep, bare-footed body stretches on the beach. The water dappled with sunbeams dancing on the surface. They seemed content, connected with each other and with the Earth.

In that moment, it dawned on me. Could living well be as simple as connecting the wisdom of our elders with what we know in the present?

My health journey

It all began when I landed in the emergency room for the first time in my life. I was having one of the most exciting moments of my career. I had launched the zero-waste fashion startup of my dreams and our company had won a massive social impact competition in Hong Kong, sending us into a whirlwind of publicity and events. As CEO, I was singly focused on growing the company at lightning speed, and I worked around the clock, running on black coffee and no sleep. I muscled through what I initially thought were minor aches and pains, with no sense of what a massive toll it was taking on my health. My body was sending me warning signs, all of which I ignored.

Since noon that day, I had been dealing with excruciating pain radiating from my midsection, which had grown considerably worse, forcing me to the hospital around midnight. It turned out that there were ulcers ripping into the entire length of my stomach wall. After spending the night in the hospital, I left with pills and instructions to take some time off work. But no matter what I did, even with the medication, I felt constantly unwell, unable to eat without pain, despite being someone who rarely fell ill, not even with a cold.

Up to this point in my life, I had never stopped to seriously consider my well-being. Growing up, I was an active tennis player, and this was enough to keep me relatively fit without having to do a lot more for my health. But through high school and college, and then business school and into parenthood, my workload continued to snowball as I took on more and gained more responsibility. I enjoyed the feeling of pushing myself to work hard and achieve. I was accustomed to pulling regular all-nighters. Whenever I was exhausted, I convinced myself that my work ethic was a badge of honor to be worn with pride. Later, I would discover that many of my friends with similar nonstop schedules had developed even more significant health issues, which had crept up on them. For many of us, health was an afterthought—there just weren't enough hours in the day to take notice of it. We were too busy working and racing toward whatever goals we had set for ourselves. But at what cost? I became distressed over my increasing reliance on medication to quell the stomach pains that disrupted my life.

As an entrepreneur, I like to figure out why things don't work. How was there such a disparity between what I thought I knew about health—particularly given the way that I was raised—and the damaging effects that my lifestyle was having on my body? In my wonderings that started from that day on the beach, it struck me that I was living on a continent where food as medicine had been a way of life for centuries. I was in the perfect place to study time-honored wellness methods first-hand, and so I decided to travel through Asia, immersing myself in the ancient longevity practices that were hidden all around me.

Asian countries consistently rank among the healthiest places in the world, and preventative self-care is their magic bullet. In 2021, Hong Kong, Macao, Japan, Korea, and Singapore dominated the top spots in the United Nations' rankings for the world's highest life expectancy rates at birth.[1] Okinawa, Japan, has long held one of the highest concentrations of centenarians in the world, with obesity running as low as single-digit rates there. And, **according to scientists from Imperial College London and the World Health Organization, in 2030, South Korea is projected to maintain the highest longevity rates in the world, outranking them all.**[2]

Due to a number of factors, including good nutrition starting in childhood and quality of healthcare, Korea's mortality rate stemming from preventable chronic conditions, like heart disease or diabetes, is estimated at a mere half of that in the United States. Its obesity rate, which is a leading risk factor in disease, is one-tenth a percentage.

While no place is perfect, these statistics offer an explanation as to why Asian countries have historically topped world health charts, and why Korea in particular offers a model for anyone seeking to boost their well-being.

Globally, Korean culture has never been more influential. In his *Guardian* article "K-Everything: The Rise and Rise of Korean Culture," journalist Tim Adams describes the phenomenon: "The world has fallen in love with everything South Korean," from K-pop music, film, and TV to K fashion, technology, and food. Growing up as a second-generation Korean American, however, I had ignored much of my Korean heritage until this point in my life. But as I spent more time in Asia and embarked on my quest, I began to uncover the wisdom of my native culture and to understand the importance of preventative self-care for good health and longevity. It was an unexpectedly delightful homecoming for me.

Ancient wisdom for wellness today

We all forget to take care of ourselves amid our busy lives. Maybe we don't get enough sleep preparing for an exam or managing a team in different time zones. Maybe we skip meals because our schedule is so crammed that we don't have the time to eat or break for lunch. Whether we are corporate types, entrepreneurs, parents, or students, we face daily hurdles that demand a lot from our bodies. Pair that with our 24/7 digital culture, and it becomes all too easy for our well-being to take a backseat, especially when everything seems just fine.

Many of us only act when we face a health problem. That was the case for me. But what if we were to fundamentally shift our thinking about the state of our health? What if, rather than being reactive, we took a proactive approach to our well-being, one that prioritized self-care? This would mean staying one step ahead of illness by encouraging the body to heal and repair itself in a continuous loop that is perfectly calibrated to our personal biology. **Rather than wait for the external signs of illness to appear—by which point it may be too late to prevent a chronic condition—we incorporate these self-care habits daily, thereby building resistance and immunity to prevent illness. As a result, we look and feel many years younger, and we have the potential to live decades longer.**

According to Google Trends, the number of searches for "self-care" has skyrocketed since the start of the COVID-19 pandemic. A Google search today yields an incredible six billion results and counting. This trending topic is often focused on women's health, but self-care is not just a fad, and it is critical across genders and age groups. Top health organizations like the Mayo Clinic and the Cleveland Clinic take a serious, health-oriented view of self-care, considering it an essential aspect to well-being; for them, self-care encompasses hygiene, nutrition, health literacy, and being body-aware enough to seek medical care when needed. Research shows that self-care leads to positive health outcomes, such as greater immunity, increased productivity, higher self-esteem, resilience, longevity, and reduced stress. Self-care is also a simple and powerful way to tackle the 70 percent of chronic illnesses that the World Health Organization deems preventable through simple lifestyle changes.

In this book, you will learn about self-care through the lens of Korean and Asian cultures, with a particular focus on interventions that date back to ancient times. These time-honored techniques encourage a preventative and proactive approach to health, and they are simple and sustainable. All are grounded in the Korean concept of yak sik dong won, which means "food is medicine," and the holistic lifestyle that revolves around this. Yak sik dong won is not about following a single, prescriptive eating plan for health, avoiding certain food groups, or adhering to restrictive protocols that can cause their own stresses;

neither is it about rejecting modern medicine. Instead, it's about opening your mind to a new way of eating and living that allows the body's natural healing systems to thrive and that works in tandem with modern healthcare advances.

Our bodies and our brains are made to work in sync, helping us to stay alive and heal at the first signs of wear and tear. But this is only possible if we encourage our natural healing process by clearing mind and body blockages, like circulation issues, and by nourishing ourselves with the right inputs: nutrient-dense foods, fluids, time, rest, movement, and emotional support from our communities. The secret lies in all the little things we do to help these along every single day.

For millennia, Korean families have passed down simple wellness knowledge from generation to generation like gifted heirlooms. But, as an increasing number of Koreans adopt a modern lifestyle, moving away from the traditional way of life, these centuries-old well-being methods are fading. I want to pass on to you these nourishing traditions, which helped to save me, and to preserve them before their healing presence slips away from our modern world. I also want to show you that making these changes is easy, sustainable, and compatible with your daily routine. Anyone can do this, whether you are living alone or with roommates, or you are a busy student or corporate executive with only moments to spare.

As I implemented the techniques and practices in this book, I was able to not only connect back to my Korean roots but also find that I was able to achieve a new kind of optimal well-being. And to my relief, I found this did not force me to reject ambitious dreams but, rather, supercharged me to continue reaching for them. Today, I am grateful to live pain-free, medication-free, and with more energy, mental clarity, and happiness than I have ever had before, even compared to my youthful twenties. In the end, I have also learned the hard way to be more kind to myself. And I finally learned to cook.

To those who are burning the candle at both ends, taxing body and mind as I once did, I will have succeeded in my mission with this book if I am able to prevent what happened to me from happening to you.

But know this first; it may seem evident, but few of us live by this truth: You will live longer and achieve more if you first take care of yourself.

SOIL

Ssukgat grows best in rich soil teeming with life. Tending to the quality of the soil is the secret to growing the most nutritious ssukgat with the brightest, loveliest colors. In much the same way, nourishing a healthy microbiome helps us humans to blossom and thrive.

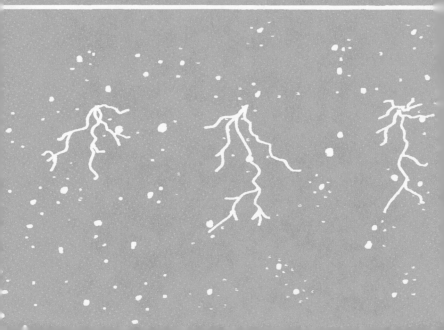

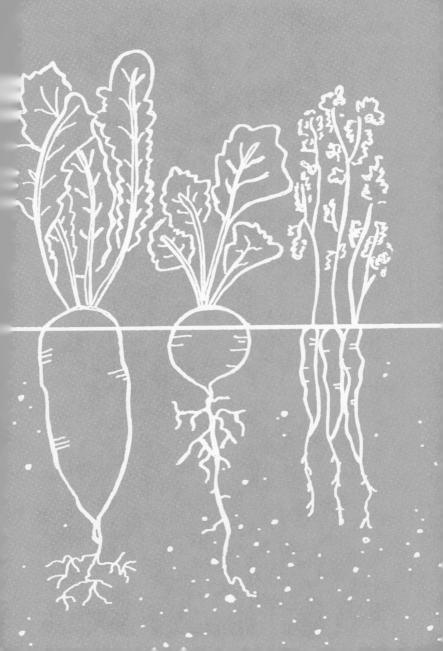

Buddhist Nuns & the Microbiome

"He that takes medicine and neglects diet wastes the skills of the physician."

—*ancient Chinese proverb*

Deep in the mountains of Naejangsan National Park in South Korea lies a secluded hermitage where Buddhist nuns live as part of a modest monastery located in the hills below. Time stands still in this verdant paradise, enveloped by a vast wood with a gurgling creek that flows and meanders, where the nuns spend their meals in reverent silence, expressing gratitude for the food spread before them. It is here that they tend to a five-hundred-year-old citrus tree that bears bitter trifoliate oranges and an unfussy garden patch where they grow Korean herbs, salad greens, chilis, eggplants, root vegetables, and other seasonal produce. They then forage for mushrooms, berries, and fruits that grow wild in the neighboring forest, practicing the ancient art of Korean temple cuisine.

The nuns are part of a hidden world that was suddenly thrust into the spotlight on Netflix for their teachings about the wonders of temple food. Although often self-taught, the nuns have inspired highly accomplished chefs to visit the monastery and learn from their naturalist philosophy on food and cooking, which they attest to being no different from pursuing their spirituality, and which also happens to be delicious. I, too, had long wanted to visit, just as I had once wanted to see the Sistine Chapel in Italy with my own eyes. Visiting the nuns was akin to seeing a living marvel in my lifetime. And like the other travelers who stayed when I did, including a chef from the famed Pujol restaurant in Mexico City and a young boxer from Portugal, I was drawn to the way these nuns breathed a next-level otherworldliness, full of happiness sans ego, all centered around something so common as home cooking. Somehow, the nuns seemed to have life figured out. Perhaps by connecting with them, we would all get a taste of that heightened sense of enlightenment for ourselves.

I visited the nuns at the start of the fall season in Korea when the leaves were turning, a sight that I did not get to see in subtropical Hong Kong, where I lived at the time. I had recently returned from the hospital and had been going through a rough patch for months, still unable to eat without grimacing in pain. By returning to Korea, I hoped to reconnect with my heritage, sensing that it held the keys to restoring my well-being. Health-promoting dishes like kimchi were central to the meals I ate as a child. But as I got older, my siblings and I adopted a modern lifestyle of convenience, and with this, fast food became part of the mix, as many of the valuable traditions that my parents brought with them from Korea began to fade away in our lives. I wanted to go back to understand how the traditions I had grown up with in my early days could be reincorporated in the daily routines of my adulthood. And as a child goes back to their mother when sick or hurt, I wanted to be close to the familiar rituals of my native heritage—to heal what I had broken.

I first heard about Korean Buddhist nuns, whose temple cuisine had inspired highly acclaimed chefs like Le Bernardin's Eric Ripert and Benu's Corey Lee, from a friend in Korea. I was intrigued by the way they prepared plant-based ingredients in their purest form yet served them in a flavorful way, and I wanted to taste and see this type of cuisine for myself. After half a day's travel from Seoul by bus, I was dropped off at the start of a long gravel path leading to a gate a mile's walk from the monastery. Once there, I dropped off my bags and set off on a walk through the bramblings of the forest to reach the nuns' remote abode.

The nuns greeted us clothed in the humble, faded attire of Buddhist habit. Little scarves around their necks, worn for protection from the wind and cold, adorned their glowing faces and freshly shaved heads, their bare skin radiant. Even with their petite frames of some four-odd

BUDDHIST NUNS & THE MICROBIOME

feet, they commanded immediate respect with their smiles, quiet confidence, and air of absolute serenity.

As the nuns began to speak, it was odd for me to hear their stream of Korean words. I had not heard my native language spoken to this extent in many years, as growing up, my parents and even my grandparents quickly conquered and took to speaking English when they were around me. For a while, though, I grew up swimming in the language at home, probably until first grade. I instinctively understood the cultural nuances and feelings that some Korean words were spoken with. At the monastery, I was pleasantly surprised that much of the language from my early memories was unlocking within me. I could read the symbols and the printed words and understand at least the basics. Through my travels in Korea, I constantly wrote and drew what I did not understand in my field notes to research later, and I re-created the dishes. These bits of knowledge became my bridge to a lost connection I was trying to rebuild. This is how I learned to be a little more Korean again.

The nuns led us into the kitchen, which, like the rest of the monastery, was extremely modest. It was a small space with a long, narrow island that took up the width of the room, an almost equally long cutting board, and just enough space for cooking burners and a sink. Simple wooden planks boarded the ceiling, walls, and floors, filling the cozy space with the pleasant aroma of cedar. Natural light spilled in through the windows, which looked out on a small working watermill set against the stunning backdrop of the Naejangsan National Park. The kitchen was stocked with well-worn clay pots; a large variety of woven baskets; huge mixing bowls, sieves, and serving plates (on the order of twenty-five inches in diameter); and small ceramic vessels filled with many small silver spoons used for measuring out various ingredients and adjusting throughout the meal preparations.

According to the nuns, if you want to know how to cook your ingredients, you must grow them from seed. Then you will know if you need to lightly boil them or eat them fresh. For these women, cooking in proximity to nature and knowing where their food comes from is a spiritual practice and a way of honoring their roots. By putting their energy into the ingredients they grow, they become one with the dishes that they create. This is part of the magic and medicine of what is plated and eaten when they cook their meals for others, and a meal is never eaten without an expression of deep gratitude. Seeing them cook, I felt like I was back in my halmoni's (grandmother's) kitchen, sitting on a stool, watching my grandmother transform ingredients from the market into a nourishing and delicious family meal. Presto. Magic.

The nuns' cooking is marked not only by their philosophical approach (putting good energy into the food, which is also why they often use bare hands to cook and mix the ingredients), but also their spontaneity as seen through constant adjustments in flavor, and ingredient pairings based on seasonality and ripeness. I learned that we call this, in Korean, uhmuni's sohn maht, a mother's intuition and discerning taste by hand, a nod to the older generation's penchant for cooking by experimentation and taste rather than closely following a recipe. The temple food was made from mostly home-grown or seasonally foraged ingredients gathered from the surrounding mountains and fields.

Persimmon trees grew wildly throughout the forest that surrounded the monastery, their fruit plucked and then strung together using a traditional method of drying and massaging to draw out the natural sugars. The result was a delicious and satisfying natural treat that was pleasantly chewy and mildly sweet. I ate these dried persimmons in the resident monastery café for visitors, which sold plant varieties in the form of coffee and teas made with berries, fruits, and medicinal roots. I tried the tea made of jujubes, vitamin-C-rich digestive Chinese dates, which cleansed my palate and complemented the sweet persimmons, all the while thinking that temple cuisine was a wellness lover's dream come true.

The healing magic of natural condiments

By tradition, these Buddhist nuns abstain from consuming animal products, with milk as an occasional exception. Because they believe that pungent spices cause digestive reactions that lessen their ability to meditate, the nuns avoid garlic, onions, chives, green onions, and leeks, five ingredients that typically serve as the foundations for flavorful cooking. How was it then that without these core aspects, they were able to make their plant-based dishes taste so delicious?

The answer, I discovered as I watched the nuns cook, was the condiments, which were discretely encased on a small lazy Susan. I found vessels for persimmon vinegar, sesame and perilla oil, and sea salt. Then there were cheong, the fermented fruit extracts that they used as natural sweeteners. These were made by macerating fruits like schisandra berries, black raspberries, and bitter trifoliate oranges and burying them in unprocessed sugars like rice grain syrup. Finally, there were the three fermented jangs, which were the most well-known in Korea—ganjang (soy sauce), gochujang (red pepper paste), and doenjang (soybean paste). The nuns were relying on these condiments to naturally add sweetness, tartness, or umami to the flavor mix.

These homemade condiments were a way to preserve natural ingredients for long periods of time and to feed the whole monastery. They were aged for decades using onggi, special earthenware made with porous structures of mountainside clay to facilitate the fermentation process and create the richest umami flavors. The nuns wouldn't touch a batch for at least three to four years, until it took on its own liquids and absorbed the healthy microbiota from the air in the forest. Rows and rows of onggi, with their glossy brown exteriors, sat together on the mountainside using centuries-old traditional techniques that were perfected over time.

The nuns kept returning to the lazy Susan, playing with different combinations to create an excitingly complex layer of flavors that bolstered their simple ingredients. This was their secret to making otherwise bland vegan cuisine come alive to the palate. The jangs and other condiments elevated the incredible freshness of the ingredients into a savory richness that made you forget you were eating vegetables. I realized, too, that the nuns were also supporting gut health and good digestion by adding these powerfully nutrient condiments to their dishes every day.

We were shown how to make four simple dishes utilizing health-boosting ingredients. The first was a mixed salad with seasonal produce including lettuces, fruits, and fresh red bell peppers, dressed with sesame seeds and natural condiments including persimmon vinegar, schisandra berry paste, wild black raspberry paste, and fermented chili paste. The second was a layered Korean radish tofu dish made in fermented soy-braised lasagna-like tiers with homemade rice grain syrup sweetener. And the last two were mushroom dishes made of king oyster and shiitake mushrooms that had been grown at the monastery. According to the nuns, the mushrooms had to be braised in the sauce—a mixture of soy, rice grain syrup, toasted sesame oil, and persimmon vinegar—until they were saturated to the core so that the inner and outer taste worked in unity.

Tasting the homemade condiments, like the nuns' incredible twenty-year soy sauce that flavored the dishes, I suddenly felt the poignancy of the moment. The jangs and other condiments were filled with the history and traditions of my Korean heritage and the memories of the many people who helped to create them. With each bite, I felt the connection to my native culture, which had come loose, growing a little stronger.

The start of my longevity pantry

Seeing that the old nuns were still so agile, with glowing, radiant skin, I was inspired to try this naturalist approach at home. Once I returned to Hong Kong, I decided that I would cook at home with my own dehydrated and preserved additions and using freshly picked, seasonal ingredients to maximize nutrition and flavor. This didn't mean that I would have to use rare or exotic ingredients or age my condiments for years as the nuns did. I knew that some of the nuns' methods just wouldn't be feasible for my busy city life. I did not have time to age salt or coddle fermented condiments for decades. I also would not be able to easily find certain ingredients that were local for them but that were not available in Hong Kong or New York, where I lived. However, I decided that I could use the same health principles, substituting more simple and attainable solutions for daily living, and still get the health benefits from the nuns' naturalist approach.

So, I set out to use all natural ingredients to make my own simple sauces, dressings, and condiments to pair with my meals. I would also aim to cook more of my meals at home with whole fruits and vegetables. And whenever I was out at a restaurant or café, I would lean more toward choosing foods with natural ingredients, making them the majority of what I ate.

Once I had decided that naturalist cooking would become the foundation of my new healthier path forward, I began to build the beginnings of a longevity pantry (see page 191). In Korean culture, yak sik also refers to a mildly sweet rice cake made to fortify with its healthy ingredients—glutinous rice, honey, pine nuts, chestnuts, and jujubes. For me, it was representative of the kind of longevity pantry that I wished to build. I went through my entire kitchen, reading nutrient labels and moving the focus away from artificial ingredients. Together with my homemade dressings, I would be able to try to avoid the refined sugars, preservatives, and high levels of sodium that often come with the packaged versions.

When I came back home from the trip, my family was amused to see me tinkering with new recipes in the kitchen. It became a habit for them to come in and ask: "What's that?" and "Can I try some?" Their curiosity fueled my energy to try different things to feed them well. It was a strange transformation that evolved over time, bit by bit, without me realizing it, until my two kids sat at dinner one day, disappointed that I hadn't tried something new on the menu. Our household was becoming a sort of casual food lab with my family members, the eager taste testers, and we all had fun trying new things together.

My first experiments in the kitchen were with persimmon vinegar, which I purchased on the internet; it's an ingredient that has proved over time to be a winning formula for food prep. A little bit goes a long way. I use it as a deliciously bright addition to leafy salads. It also works well as a milder and more nutritious substitute for apple cider vinegar tonics used for their metabolism boosting, antibacterial properties and blood sugar management to be taken before meals. Just dilute a small spoon of the vinegar with a dash of water. I started to remember the vinegar uses from my childhood, that, for instance, naengmyeon, the cold buckwheat noodles my mother served in ice-cold brine, tastes better and is more nutritious if you add vinegar and hot mustard to the soup. I studied all the possible vinegars to use at home, and I discovered that this category of food increases metabolism and with practically no calories. To date, I have added the following vinegars as staples in my pantry:

Persimmon vinegar: This remains my favorite vinegar to use for its mild and sweet taste, and it now sits on top of my counter at all times. I use a tablespoon diluted with a bit of water as a health tonic, before tucking into meals, and also as a finishing splash for soups. It also supports the heart, liver, skin, and digestive health and has more vitamin C, vitamin A, and potassium than the more well-known apple cider vinegar.

Black vinegar: I encountered this vinegar through my travels; I mix it with a bit of soy sauce to make a simple and flavorful dip for dumplings.

White vinegar: I use this neutral-flavored vinegar to add acidity to many of my dishes and in a DIY spray (filling a spray bottle with three parts water to one part vinegar) to clean produce prior to a final rinse with cold water. Studies show that a vinegar rinse can remove pesticides and kill up to 98 percent of bacteria.

Rice wine vinegar: Used ubiquitously in Asian cooking, this vinegar lends a mildly sweet flavor.

Apple cider vinegar: This acidic-tasting vinegar contains chlorogenic acid—which boosts our health defenses and metabolism—from the apples that it is made with. It is the vinegar most commonly found in wellness kitchens.

Balsamic vinegar: In combination with olive oil as a simple dressing or dip, this vinegar that has long been part of the Mediterranean diet is sweet and contains resveratrol—which helps to reduce LDL cholesterol (the bad kind)—from the grapes that are used to make it.

After seeing the nuns' use of fresh fruits and healthier natural sweeteners, I overhauled this entire category in my pantry, too. I replaced my white sugar—which I found to be linked to my afternoon energy dips—with less processed and more nutritious alternatives like bee pollen, maple syrup, vanilla extract, and honey. I switched out sugary drinks for water or tea made with ingredients like fresh mint leaves. I started using fruits like dates, raisins, and cranberries in my cooking. And I replaced the artificial sweetener I had been putting in my morning coffee with monk fruit extract in a dropper that I'd bought in a health food store or I skipped sweetener altogether.

When it came to procuring the more difficult-to-source ingredients that I had learned about from the nuns, I was able to find many of them online in powdered or otherwise dried form, including schisandra and jujube berries and capsicum-rich, metabolism-boosting chilis. Using dried and dehydrated foods as ingredients at home was a big shift, with the added benefit that the dried versions lasted longer and were ready to use once I reconstituted them with water. I found that these dried versions also capture the ingredients at their peak state of ripeness.

I discovered a replacement for the nuns' age-coddled salt and fermented condiments in store-bought pink Himalayan salt, which contains eighty-four other minerals and trace elements and has a nice delicate taste, as well as coarse sea salt. Both are derived from seawater and are less processed than table salt, thereby retaining more nutrients. Korean store-bought fermented condiments like gochujang were part of my previous vernacular, but I began to use these in meals with renewed interest.

After making these adjustments to my pantry, I focused on the cooking. As I was learning more about our cultural recipes, I kept calling my parents to ask how to cook them. For any Korean American learning how to make their heritage food, there are the usual nebulous instructions from Korean parents without measurements. Take rice, for instance. "First, place your hand flat on top of the uncooked rice, then fill rice cooker with enough water to cover the top of your hand." When I learned about the intuitive sohn maht method of discerning the recipe by taste, I understood that this was just how it was done with the older generations and how the newer ones were learning. I stopped stressing about following recipes to a tee and started to consider how I wanted the food to taste. And sometimes I adapted them to include new methods and ingredients supported by the new health science I was learning to utilize more.

Cooking became a more casual and creative affair that involved tasting and riffing. Like the nuns, I cooked with bare hands and no recipes. I focused on trying to appreciate the simple quality, basic texture, and flavor of each ingredient. I became more mindful of the way I was cooking and eating, paying attention to flavor and texture. If I wanted to add more crunch to a salad, I would add cucumber or some nuts. If I was craving more sweetness in a dressing, I would add homemade applesauce. To make it more savory, I would add soy sauce. Lemons, too, became part of my every day after seeing the nuns use citrus fruits regularly; I would add a squeeze of it to everything for a bit of acidity and the added vitamin C. Food preparation became like creating a painting that became more complex as I gained confidence and added more layers of flavor over time. Cooking became one of my favorite activities, reinforced every time I was greeted with joy after presenting a home-cooked meal to loved ones.

In the past, I had rarely cooked for myself, but now that old version of me seemed unrecognizable. My cooking at home wasn't elaborate, but it was healthy, efficient, and nourishing, just what I needed to maintain my well-being within my busy life.

Building what I began to think of as my longevity pantry is a practice that continues to evolve and grow as I discover and research new ingredients. It was the first of many steps that I took toward transforming my health. Inspired by the Buddhist nuns, I had begun a resolute shift to eat more naturally every day.

Rediscovering the benefits
of fermentation

Dating back to Neolithic China (7000–6600 BCE), long before the advent of refrigeration, our ancestors used the natural process of fermentation to preserve food. This was done in early forms of earthenware dug fully or partially underground to prepare for winters when food couldn't be grown or to save vegetables that were past their prime. Along the way, they discovered that fermentation was also a method for making foods taste better.

When I learned that fermentation had origins in ancient China, I decided to visit Chengdu, the capital of southwestern China's Sichuan province and home of the Chuançais Museum, which is devoted to showcasing the history of fermentation and Sichuan cuisine. The museum's large cobblestone courtyard, surrounded by an exotic garden of giant fronds and ginkgo trees, featured two hundred vats of chili beans, proudly hailed as the "soul of Sichuan cuisine." I walked the halls of the museum and learned how Chinese cuisine developed its complexity over numerous dynasties and as new ingredients were introduced through trade on the Silk Road, such as South American hot chilis, which were later reinterpreted for Chinese and Korean ferments to great effect. As I pressed my nose to the glass to gaze at the collections of intricately painted pickling pots, which ranged from the oxidized and primitive to the exquisitely restored, I marveled at the fact that I was seeing original fermentation relics. This was proof that fermentation had been invented and mastered as a way of survival so many centuries ago. I was only now discovering its benefits.

Fermentation was one of the key techniques used by the nuns. They mainly used two natural and healthy food preparations for their produce: dehydration—drying ingredients with sunshine or under shade,

How fermentation leads to much more

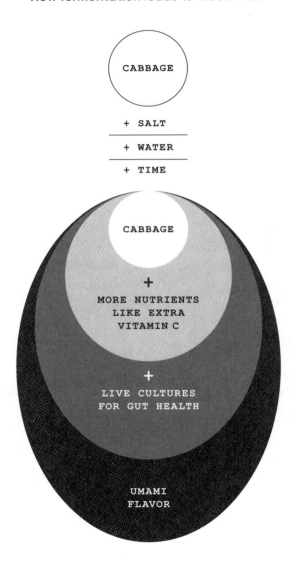

CABBAGE

+ SALT

+ WATER

+ TIME

CABBAGE

+

MORE NUTRIENTS
LIKE EXTRA
VITAMIN C

+

LIVE CULTURES
FOR GUT HEALTH

UMAMI
FLAVOR

blanching then drying them; and preservation—by pickling, fermenting, or making cheong, their fruit extracts. Pickling involves soaking foods in an acidic liquid like vinegar. Cheong, a traditional medicinal food in Korea, is made by extracting fruits and plants, then combining them with honey or sugar. While both pickling and cheong are healthy, it's the fermentation, as with kimchi or jangs, that results in the live probiotics that are particularly beneficial for gut healing.

Fermentation breaks down a food's molecular structure, a process that helps preserve the food and makes it more digestible and nutritious. Before people had the ability to keep foods fresh with refrigeration, fermentation was a practical solution for storing these foods over a length of time.

Fermentation may be the simplest way of preserving food, requiring no heat or cooking, while simultaneously maximizing the nutritional profile of your diet. Fermented foods go through a transformation from one type of food to another by way of bacteria, yeasts, or other microorganisms. When we take a fermenting agent, like yeast, sugar, or salt, and let it sit on ingredients without exposure to oxygen, we feed healthful bacteria that in turn help our bodily functions when ingested. For example, when we ferment a cabbage with salt, the sugars from the cabbage convert into lactic and acetic acids that create an environment for the good bacteria to grow, bacteria that we later eat when we consume the fermented cabbage. Cabbage becomes sauerkraut or kimchi, soybeans turn into miso or natto, and milk can be made into yogurt and cheeses.

In the nineteenth century, renowned French biologist, microbiologist, and chemist Louis Pasteur discovered, among other breakthroughs, the concept of pasteurization, a heating method to treat bacterial contamination in beverages like milk and wine, a discovery that saved many lives. Subsequently microorganisms tended to be cast as a dark shadow in medicine, as it was understood that germs caused diseases, and this led to a focus on sterilization and hyper cleanliness to kill germs. Years later, science would discover the flip side of Pasteur's concept of bacteria—that there are beneficial health effects to be gained from nurturing your good bacteria, not just killing the bad.

There are numerous benefits to eating naturally fermented foods (NFFs), but only if the beneficial bacteria are kept alive. Read labels and look for products that are "traditionally brewed" or "naturally fermented," rather than those that have been heated from pasteurization, baking, filtering, or making a product shelf stable, all of which can kill good bacteria. NFFs contain the magic combination of digestive enzymes (which help us to break down foods); probiotics (live beneficial bacteria that support the digestive process); prebiotics (nondigestible foods that feed our probiotic population); and synbiotics (the by-product when prebiotics and probiotics combine).

NFFs have an increased bioactive and bioavailable nutrient profile that your system can easily absorb, more effectively supporting the digestive system and ultimately our immune system than supplements can. Research has also shown that fermentation can increase B and C vitamins and a range of enhanced nutrients like omega-3 fatty acids in the food, eliminate antinutrients (that make grains indigestible, for example), and inhibit foodborne pathogens. Healthy NFFs with probiotics include kimchi, sauerkraut, unpasteurized miso, live culture olives, kefir drinks, red wine, beet kvass, and kombucha.

Finally, the umami flavor that results from fermentation makes vegetables taste deliciously savory, and it's one of the secrets of Korean cuisine. Umami tends to amplify the other flavors, and its richness is found in fermented condiments like doenjang (fermented soybean paste) as well as foods like mushrooms, anchovies, and caramelized onions. By embracing fermentation, we can eat more like the Buddhist nuns, and with a lot more flavor too.

Behold the humble cabbage

For anyone growing up in a Korean household, spicy fermented cabbage—kimchi—is a star, superfood ingredient that can make an appearance at breakfast, lunch, and dinner. Korea has hundreds of varieties of kimchi, which increase in assortment when the cabbage is cultivated and coddled for age, fermentation, and spiciness. Nowadays, there are even special kimchi refrigerators that replicate the cold underground conditions of the past, the way kimchi had been traditionally stored. For many Koreans, kimchi is central to their culinary identity and brings recollections of kimjang, a fall tradition of making and sharing kimchi as a community. After all, it was kimchi, with its ability to be preserved for long durations, that fed the nation through the harshest winters.

Cabbage plays an important role in the Korean diet for its versatility and health benefits. There are four hundred kinds of cabbage, including red, white, cauliflower, broccoli, savoy, napa, kohlrabi, bok choy, choi sum, kale, and Romanesco broccoli. It is full of vitamin U, a little known compound, not technically a vitamin, that is highly available in raw cabbage juice. Vitamin U has shown indications of protecting and strengthening the mucous membrane of the gastrointestinal lining, thus a potential antidote to peptic ulcers. In a series of studies, Dr. Garnett Cheney at Stanford University's School of Medicine explored the antiulcer factor of vitamin U. In one study, he found that after administering raw cabbage juice to thirteen patients, the healing time for seven who had duodenal ulcers was 10.4 days, compared with the standard average of 37 days, while six of those patients with gastric ulcers healed in 7.3 days, compared with the average 42 days.[1] In another study involving ninety-two patients, Dr. Cheney found 61 percent of this group to be pain-free within four days, while 86 percent of the patients were pain-free within two weeks. Cabbage is also part of the cruciferous family that contains sulforaphane, which are antioxidants that cancel free radicals that weaken and damage healthy cells.

Both kimchi and sauerkraut utilize the humble cabbage as a base vegetable. Once I discovered its benefits, I added more cabbage to my diet. I began regularly drinking a bit of cabbage juice (which tastes mildly bitter) as an effective natural remedy for my ulcers, along with using cabbage leaves, gently steamed, to make wraps. Within two weeks, I was able to build up my stomach health again. Cabbage has since become a staple on my grocery list, and I never go without it.

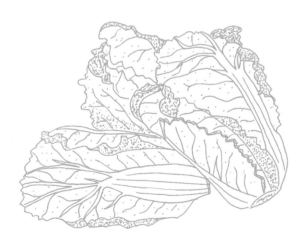

Everyday sauerkraut

One delicious way to have a little more cabbage every day is to eat it fermented as a small side dish with each meal. Enter sauerkraut, the tangy, no-spice cousin of kimchi. This recipe is sauerkraut pared down to its simplest form, and it's easy to make on a regular basis. In fact, at its roots, kimchi is more about preservation than spice. Prior to spice being added, kimchi was just a sour fermented cabbage and much closer to sauerkraut in its ancestry. Both high-quality sauerkraut and kimchi are increasingly available in supermarkets these days if you don't feel like making this at home.

INGREDIENTS

Makes 1½ quarts

1 cabbage, 3 pounds, cored and shredded

1½ tablespoons sea salt or pink Himalayan salt

1 tablespoon caraway seeds (optional)

METHOD

1. Place the shredded cabbage in a large bowl and pound it with a wooden pounder or pestle tool to release its juice. Mix in the salt (the salt and the cabbage juice will create a brine). Add the caraway seeds, if using, and thoroughly mix.

2. Pack everything firmly into a 2-quart mason jar, pressing your ingredients down and compressing out all the air. The cabbage must be fully submerged in the liquid. Cover tightly and keep at room temperature for about 3 days. Watch for bubbling, a sign of fermentation and an indicator that the sauerkraut is ready. You'll have live bacteria, probiotics, and a superfood filled with vitamins that will keep refrigerated for up to 6 months.

Nabak kimchi (water kimchi)

This is a refreshing kimchi of young cabbage leaves and radish in a tangy broth. As the kimchi continues to ferment, over time the broth will taste tangier. Some of my friends even drink small amounts of the broth for natural electrolytes and probiotics. Because of its clean taste, restaurants will often use this dish as a palate cleanser and flavor it with pine nuts, whole chilis, or bae (Korean pear). Without the fish sauce or salted shrimp often used in making traditional kimchi recipes, this dish is vegan too. I typically make half this amount for my household.

Recipe note

Kimchi is meant to be eaten in relatively small amounts, as a side dish or a topping, to accompany your meals. Too many fermented foods, especially for the uninitiated, can cause bloating as the good bacteria gets rid of the bad, but you can slowly build up the amount you consume over time to avoid the bloating. Kimchi-style fermentation, with its spicy seasonings, can also be applied to many other ingredients, like perilla leaves, eggplant, mushrooms, cucumber, oysters, soybean sprouts, pumpkin, octopus, burdock root, tomatoes, and even sweet fruits like apples.

INGREDIENTS

Makes 1 gallon

1 mu (Korean radish; see page 41), 1.5 pounds, unpeeled, quartered, then thinly sliced

1 napa cabbage, 1 pound, cut into similar-sized pieces as the radish

4 tablespoons sea salt or pink Himalayan salt, divided

1½ tablespoons gochugaru (red chili flakes)

2 tablespoons minced garlic

Slices of bae (Korean pear), ginger, apple, or cucumber; pine nuts; and/or whole chilis for garnish (optional)

METHOD

1. In a large bowl, combine the radish, cabbage, and 2 tablespoons of the salt, tossing gently by hand. Let sit for about 30 minutes, until the cabbage is wilted.

2. In a separate large bowl, dissolve the remaining 2 tablespoons salt in 10 cups filtered water. Place the gochugaru and garlic in a cheesecloth and squeeze it in the water several times. Remove the cheesecloth.

3. Pour the brine over the radish and cabbage and stir well to combine.

4. Pack everything firmly into a clean 1 gallon mason jar, pressing the ingredients down and pressing out all the air. Cover tightly and keep at room temperature for about 2 days, then move to the refrigerator. Eat it within 3 weeks of making it.

5. To serve, ladle the kimchi with broth into a bowl. Top with bae, apples, or cucumbers to add a crunchy texture and/or naturally sweet taste that pairs well with the kimchi brine. Garnish with bae, ginger apple, cucumber, pine nuts, and/or whole chilis, if using.

Microbiome health: Where modern science meets ancient wisdom

A most simple and effective way to take charge of your health and to prevent disease is by embracing the naturalist eating principles favored by the nuns. Modern science has begun to support this traditional eating approach, which contributes to a healthy microbiome and builds gut resilience. While gut-friendly foods, like those that are fermented, have early origins, scientific study of how they benefit the microbiome has exploded in the twenty-first century. This has led to great leaps like the Human Microbiome Project, and healthy bacteria derived from foods for effective self-care has become a buzzing area in medicine.

Your microbiome lives throughout your body, including your mouth; it is the ecosystem of microorganisms—the bacteria, fungi, and viruses, that exist within your body. It controls your metabolism and digestion by helping you to break down your food; supplies essential nutrients; affects your mood, as 90 percent of your serotonin receptors are located in the gut; and deeply affects your immunity (and pathogen fighting power), as 70 percent of your immune system resides in the gut.

The things you do to feed and cultivate your microbiome affect the bacterial balance in your microbiome, playing an essential role in how healthy you are and how you feel on a day-to-day basis. Gut health is about having more friendly bacteria than harmful bacteria in the microbiome that exists in your gut. Based on a growing body of research, we know that a healthy functioning gut can lead to numerous benefits, including radiant skin, mental clarity, weight control, and physical energy. In their book *The Hidden Half of Nature*,[2] David R. Montgomery and Anne Biklé reveal why nurturing healthy microbiomes can transform both medicine and agriculture. Through a fascinating account of experiences in reviving their barren yard and recovering from a health

> **Gardening for your gut**
> - Forest bathe
> - Have contact with diverse vegetation and dirt
> - Eat mindfully. Try using chopsticks to slow your pace. Remember to chew your food to aid digestion and allow your mind the twenty minutes it needs to send signals of fullness
> - Eat mostly plant-based foods
> - Eat foods with fiber
> - Eat fermented foods to boost friendly bacteria in your gut
> - Use natural sweeteners, which don't feed harmful bacteria, which leads to sugar cravings
> - Move your body daily

crisis, the authors drew incredible parallels linking how **both plants and humans thrive when we cultivate beneficial microbes in both.**

A healthy microbiome is increasingly being linked to the prevention, reversal, and even eradication of a host of chronic diseases, from obesity to neurodegenerative diseases. According to gut experts, **you are only as healthy as your gut bacteria**. A growing body of scientists believe that microbial diversity within your body is a key factor that determines who survives potentially deadly viruses, and with this, food is emerging as the most influential factor, since the bacteria residing within us feed from and thrive on the food that we eat. So, it's important to do things to feed the garden of your gut and digestion; they impact more than you would think.

Researchers suggest taking the measures listed above to help support friendly bacteria and improve your microbiome. When you take care of your gut microbiome, planting healthy bacteria through eating a plant diverse diet, the good bacteria will stick around to support you. If you neglect it, for example feeding the toxic bacteria that feed on a diet high in sugars, the good bacteria and their immune-supporting powers will leave the garden of your gut.

Though the science on the microbiome is relatively new, remarkably, the nuns have been holding the keys to the microbiome and well-being all along. With temple food, it's all about supporting digestion while simultaneously feeding the mind, soul, and body to achieve harmony. For the nuns, it is not just about what you eat, but how you eat it.

You can improve your microbiome in a single day

Even when we are out of balance, the good news is that by making simple lifestyle and dietary changes, we can immediately rectify, or at least significantly improve, our microbiome health. In a 2014 study conducted at the University of Pittsburgh, scientists set out to understand why African Americans had rates of colon cancer that were twelve times higher than rural South Africans.[3] For a mere two weeks, the researchers effectively swapped the diets of twenty African Americans (previously high in fat intake with meat and cheese) and twenty South Africans (on a traditional African diet, high in fiber and low in fat, with little meat and plenty of vegetables, beans, and cornmeal). They found that even within this short period of time, the participants' microbiomes altered considerably. Those on the traditional African diet increased the production of butyrate, a fatty acid proven to protect against colon cancer, while those on the American diet developed biomarkers in their gut that were presets for cancer. Perhaps more fascinating, according to scientists at Harvard and the University of California, large microbial shifts can occur within the body in as little as twenty-four hours, demonstrating the remarkable flexibility of our human response to diet. A change in the way you eat can make all the difference.

A happy gut calls for digestive aids

Promoting good digestion is central to the nuns' cooking and eating philosophy. As I dug deeper, I recognized that they were preparing every single item on their menu to be easy on the gut. In addition to fermented foods, their diets were rich in other elements that boosted digestion, including prebiotics from mushrooms and seaweed; warm liquids like soups, teas, and warm water; a wide range of seasonal, fiber-rich fruits and vegetables; and digestion-boosting vinegars.

Their plant-based dishes were all anti-inflammatory, too, balancing out the naturally acidic environment in the stomach. And beyond what they were eating, there was also a symbiosis with the healthy microbiota in their natural environment, as they spent hours outdoors in the forest and in their garden each day. I would observe this sort of active time spent outdoors time and time again during my travels across Asia, and I would learn, to my surprise, that this is also crucial to cultivating a healthy and happy gut.

Supporting good digestion is incredibly important to our health. Your stomach has its own tools for breaking down foods—gastric acid and digestive enzymes—but you can aid the process by eating like the nuns do. Digestion is a process that requires more energy than any other internal function of the human body, and experts estimate that half or more of your total energy is actually focused on digestion. When you eat foods that aid digestion, you help your body to divert more energy to other bodily processes that optimize functioning, including cell repair and nutrient absorption.

In Korean culture, digestive aids include fruits, which are highly effective in breaking down protein and used as a simple remedy for stomach problems. Kiwi and bae are used as both natural sweeteners and tenderizers for kalbi (beef short ribs). Papayas are also used in many Asian cuisines as a natural means to tenderize meat before cooking.

The reverence of fruit in Asia

Some modern health trends veer toward an avoidance of fruits because of their sugar content. However, whole, fresh fruits with the peel and unsweetened natural dried fruits are different from concentrated fruit juices, which can be laden with sugar without the fiber, and play an incredibly important role in Asia's food culture. Fruits are revered in the Asian culture for their nutritional profile, with their powerful combination of prebiotics, digestive enzymes, and natural sweetness. They are considered delicacies, eaten at breakfast, as a snack, after dinner, and even presented as gifts of well-being, thoughtfully encased in a tradi-

---

Fruits with digestive enzymes
- **Papaya, pineapple, kiwi, fig, bae (Korean pear):** Contain protease, which breaks down protein
- **Mango, ripe banana:** Contain amylase, which breaks down carbs and is also present in saliva
- **Avocado:** Contains lipase, which breaks down fats
- **Unripe banana, jackfruit:** Contain prebiotics, a digestive aid not produced by the body

---

tional Korean bojagi, an eco-friendly way to wrap a gift with reusable fabric.

In Korea, perfectly grown golden pineapples, replete with a full crown of green spikes, and ping-pong-sized ruby grapes packaged in jewelry box–like containers serve as thoughtful gifts for special occasions like a housewarming or for an employer. In Japan, watermelons are grown into heart shapes or cubed to fit in refrigerators. In China, pears are grown in the molds of Buddhas and little babies. Harvesting beautiful fruits can be a sport in Asia, sometimes warranting luxury price tags of thousands of dollars for perfectly grown melons or tennis-ball-sized strawberries.

Along hiking trails in Korea, food stalls selling crispy cucumbers, steamed corn on the cob, and sweet potatoes provide a natural pick-me-up for weary hikers trying to reach the summit. And every night in places like Chengdu, China, portable bicycle fruit stalls with red lamps are pedaled throughout the city for those craving a late-night snack. In Korea and across Asia, it is common to see fresh fruits sold in public spaces like parks, train stations, bus depots, and directly on trains. It is also common in Asia to find public spaces lined with an impressive load of fruit trees, and families will grow smaller varieties in their home backyards, where they can pluck the fruits at their perfect seasonal peak.

Fruit ideas

For anyone making the switch to a more natural lifestyle, fruits should play a part. They help us get a daily dose of colorful antioxidants, and they are a great source of hydration and digestive enzymes. If you worry about the natural sugar content in fruits, I encourage you to eat them whole and with the peel and avoid juicing them. The fiber, from both the inner fruit and peel, slows down the absorption of a fruit's natural sugars into the bloodstream. Eating fruits whole will also make you feel fuller and encourage you to eat them in moderation. And if you're a person who doesn't love vegetables, fruits can be a great source of fiber in your daily diet. Below are some of my favorite fruit ideas from my travels and learnings.

Pineapple

Fresh pineapples contain living bromelain enzyme, which helps to break down food. Pineapple is great as a snack and can act as a powerful digestive aid, especially on an empty stomach. Eating raw pineapple is an easy way to get more fiber and manganese, a mineral that supports stronger bones and connective tissue.

Cucumber

Raw cucumber is a great portable snack, super-hydrating with 96 percent water content, and packed with vitamin K. Cucumbers are great for your skin, and they are particularly good as a snack if you are trying to control your weight. Try them chilled from the refrigerator to help your body cool down in hot temperatures. I like eating them dipped in savory Korean condiments like ssamjang, a fermented chili and bean paste, and I prepare them in an easy pickled recipe called oi muchim in Korean, mixing a teaspoon of salt, a teaspoon of minced garlic, a teaspoon of toasted sesame oil, a splash of rice vinegar, and a sprinkle of gochugaru (red pepper flakes), rice vinegar, and sesame seeds. (Although the classic recipe calls for squeezing out the water naturally found in cucumbers, I like to keep this in.)

Pears

Freshly grated bae (Asian pear) makes a fresh, crispy topper to cold noodles. Bae is also especially good for marinating meat, adding a naturally sweet flavor. Pears are known to be good for the lungs and have digestive enzymes to help you break down your meal. Like apples, pears also contain chlorogenic acid, which boosts your metabolism. I like to eat all sorts of pears, including bae and Bosc pears.

Tangerines

Tangerines have long been present in South Korea and were often presented to Korean royalty, their peels dried and aged to use in herbal medicine for teas and often bestowed as gifts in crates. Koreans like to give one another wellness gifts, in food, teas, and beauty, as a sign of love.

Stone fruits

Studies have shown that stone fruits, including cherries, peaches, and plums, are rich in anthocyanins, which may offer protection against cancer.[4] Apricots and mangoes are rich in beta-carotene. Stone fruits, like plums, are portable and very easy to incorporate into your routine at a more budget-friendly price.

Watermelon

Watermelon is 92 percent water, which aids in hydration. Studies have shown eating watermelon to be waist-shrinking, to aid in weight loss, and to lower bad cholesterol. Like tomatoes, watermelon contains a special ingredient within its red flesh called lycopene, which increases metabolism and protects DNA. Scientists have also proposed that lycopene can inhibit cancer cell growth, prevent DNA damage, and enhance enzymes that break down cancer-causing compounds. Watermelon—and tomatoes in all forms and fresh with balsamic vinegar and salt—are on heavy rotation for me when they are in season in the summer.

Keep a seasonal fruit bowl within reach

Place a bowl or platter of colorful fruit right on your kitchen or dining table. I began this change to encourage my kids to try new produce, like the delicious kiwi berry, and to reach for these fruits if they were hungry in between meals. It's been a great way to have easy access to a quick snack, along with a visual reminder to eat our fruits. It's also been a great way to bring a little nature into our home.

Steamed kabocha squash

Kabocha squash is highly nutritious, offering a spectrum of vitamins contained within its green outer skin, bright orange inner flesh, and seeds. High in fiber and low in carbs, the kabocha's glycemic index is relatively low, so it won't spike your blood sugar levels. Steamed, it tastes like a deliciously sweet chestnut, and its soft, digestible skin adds a boost of fiber. I also like to eat it as a snack or side dish with a little maple syrup.

Recipe notes

If you only have a small pot, you can slice the kabocha and steam for 8 to 13 minutes, but note that it's much harder to cut into the tough skin of a raw kabocha.

You can roast the seeds for a flavorful and healthy snack. After cleaning, drying, and seasoning the seeds with your choice of spices like gochugaru (red chili flakes) or cinnamon, roast at 350°F for 12 to 15 minutes, until they give off a nutty aroma. Eating whole kabocha seeds provides fiber, an excellent source of zinc from the shells, and nutrients like iron.

INGREDIENTS

Serves 6

1 kabocha squash, 2 pounds

METHOD

1. Steam the entire kabocha, skin-on, in an Instant Pot on high pressure for 10 minutes, or in a big pot with steamer basket for 20 minutes, until the flesh is easily pierced with a fork.

2. Slice into bitesized pieces, which is easiest along the spine, before serving.

3. It can be stored in the refrigerator for up to 4 days.

Healing mushroom broth

This broth is ideal for sipping throughout the day and through a cold. This recipe, which I adapted from the Buddhist nuns, is now a household favorite, and I make it all the time as a main course for lunch with sides or as a side dish to the main course. The mushrooms have a nice chewy texture, in contrast to the clear broth that has a kick from the ginger and chili flakes. A delicious umami flavor is achieved with mushrooms and kombu, an important ingredient in the base broth of many Korean recipes.

Recipe notes

Purchasing mushrooms in dried form gives you access to high-quality mushrooms that are not always found fresh in grocery stores, like shiitake mushrooms, which are prized for their rich umami taste and their many health benefits, including boosting immunity.

Mushrooms have immunological properties and have been used for centuries in Asia. The nuns like to use the more exotic mushrooms that they forage in their surrounding forests, such as black trumpet and shingled hedgehog mushrooms, but cooking with varieties like shiitake and maitake are also great for staying healthy during cold and flu season. Fresh mushrooms like cremini, portobello, button, or oyster mushrooms could also be added.

Chilis are rich in capsicum, a great source of vitamin C, vitamin A, and antioxidants. Red chilis contain more capsicum than green ones.

Lemons can add additional vitamin C and a flavorful acidic balance to the soup.

INGREDIENTS

Serves 2

3 slices ginger

1 cup kongnamul (soybean sprouts)

6 small dried shiitake mushrooms

6 dried jujubes, sliced

1-inch piece of kombu

1 dried red chili

½ mu (Korean radish), 0.75 lb, quartered lengthwise, then thinly sliced

2 tablespoons gukganjang (Korean soup soy sauce) or other naturally brewed soy sauce

Sea salt or pink Himalayan salt

A dash of vinegar or a squeeze of lemon, for finishing (optional)

METHOD

1. Scrub the ginger and keep its skin on. Rinse the kongnamul. Rinse the shiitakes, jujubes, kombu, and chili and then soak them in a small bowl with ½ cup filtered water for 20 minutes. Strain, keeping the soaking water for the stock base. Cut the reconstituted shiitakes and the chili into thin slices.

2. Place the jujube, chili, kombu, and ginger slices in a medium pot with 3½ cups filtered water and bring to a boil over high heat. Add the sliced mushrooms and radish.

3. Season with the gukganjang. Add the kongnamul, bring the soup to a boil once more, and boil for 3 to 5 minutes, until the kongnamul breaks down a bit to become translucent.

4. Carefully remove and discard the kombu and ginger before serving. Add salt to taste and a dash of vinegar or a squeeze of lemon juice for acidity, if desired, as the last step before serving.

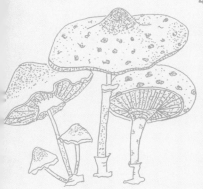

A nun's care for the common cold

Some of the nuns refrained from dining with us at the monastery because they were observing a twenty-eight-day fast. However, following the meal, they nimbly scaled the cleaned countertop to sit with crossed legs in front of us and lead us in a smiling meditation. Their agility and strength surprised and delighted me. I would later observe this in many of the seniors I met throughout my travels in Asia. The nuns asked us to reflect on the food that we had just eaten—what went into growing the food and cooking it, and how this food would now transform and become part of us, shaping our minds and body, as we left the temple and returned to our homes across the globe.

Before I left the nuns, I asked them what happens when people get sick in the monastery and whether they had any cold or flu remedies to share. They explained that they do not take over-the-counter cold medicines, because no matter what is done, it takes seven to ten days to recover, and therefore it is better not to pollute the body with unnecessary medicines. Instead, they believe in allowing the body to heal itself first. The nuns also concentrate on easy-to-digest foods while they are sick, like juk, as my parents had done, and they drink a healing mushroom broth (see page 34) to help support the recovery period. I thanked them for sharing their special wisdom with me and hugged their diminutive figures, marveling how so much wisdom could be housed within these gentlewomen.

The Whole Plant: A Zero-Waste Approach

"Cutting food waste is a delicious way of saving money,
helping to feed the world and protect the planet."

—*Tristram Stuart, environmental and food waste activist*

If you were to grow a plant in your own garden, or forage in the wild like the Buddhist nuns do, you would witness its full blossoming from top to bottom. You would watch it grow from seed to the height of its maturation, until you plucked it at just the right moment, when it was at its most ripe and delicious. It would take the plant time to get to this state, and as you waited, you might consider the ways to use the plant in its entirety, not wasting any of the gifts that nature has provided. This is the naturalist mindset that started long ago in Korea, and I refer to it as the zero-waste or whole plant approach.

Whole plant eating means fully utilizing what has grown, even if imperfectly shaped, and using as much of the plant as possible from top to bottom, inside and out, including the peel, top leaves, stalks, and roots. Eating the whole plant means not throwing anything away. In doing so, you not only avoid waste and strain on your wallet, but you also benefit from the nutrients that are otherwise lost when these peels, leaves, and roots are trimmed off and discarded. Eating the whole plant was a way of life for my ancestors, who used different parts of the plants for natural medicine. As a side note, they also apply this same concept to using the whole animal, which is why it is common to see pigs' feet, organs, and other animal parts not typical of a Western menu. The idea is that nothing gets wasted.

Ugly produce is good for you

When you shop for produce in a modern grocery store, you will find fruit that has been selected for perfection and apples that have been polished to a high shine. However, researchers have found that eating the blemished parts of plants can actually be more nutritious. Root vegetables that are oddly shaped or twisted or otherwise "imperfect" plants are just as nutritious as their perfect mirrors. This includes peels, skins, rinds, and fruits and vegetables that are bruised. Scarred Braeburn apple peels have been found to have one to four times more antioxidant activity than unblemished peels.[1] Scientists posit that the visible scars on unbroken skin can be signs of additional nutrition yielded through successful battles with pests, battles that release more antioxidants as a natural defense mechanism. As part of your toolbox for natural prevention, ugly plants shouldn't be discarded.

Edible peels, when scrubbed and washed properly, may be the most underrated part of fruits and vegetables. They are often the most nutritious part of the plant. Peels are rich in fiber, vitamins, minerals, and antioxidants, and consuming the peel is an easy way to boost your total intake of nutrients. Consider this: A raw apple with skin contains up to 267 percent more vitamin K, 50 percent more vitamin A, 15 per-

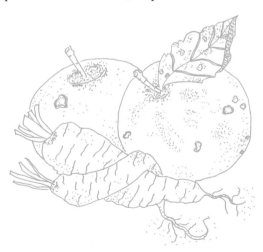

cent more vitamin C, 20 percent more calcium, and up to 19 percent more potassium than a peeled apple.[2] A boiled potato, with skin, can contain up to 76 percent more vitamin C, 16 percent more potassium, 11 percent more folate, and 10 percent more magnesium and phosphorus than a peeled one;[3] up to 31 percent of the total amount of fiber in a vegetable can be found in its skin.[4] Antioxidant levels can be up to 328 times higher in fruit peels than in the pulp.[5] One study even found that removing peach skin results in almost 50 percent fewer antioxidants.[6] And the list goes on.

What then to do with edible peels? When washed, you can eat the skins of pears, apples, even kiwis, cucumber, eggplant, tomatoes, and stone fruit (e.g., peaches and plums), root vegetables (e.g., baked potatoes, parsnips, and carrots) and on squashes (e.g., steamed pumpkin and zucchini). You can also grate citrus fruits like lemons, oranges, and limes and freeze the zest for cooking or for steeping tea. Peels can also be added to smoothies, sauces, and stir-fries to boost nutrients. And you can make some of them into healthy chips. At home, I always ask, "And have you eaten the skin?"

Likewise, I also don't throw out root ends, top leaves, or outer leaves, which are often more nutritious than the main plant and delicious additions to cooking. Beet greens, which have been used for medicinal purposes since ancient times, are loaded with carotenes and minerals, such as calcium, iron, magnesium, phosphorous, vitamins C, E, B_6, B_1, B_2, B_3, and folate and have multiple cleansing effects on the liver, digestive system, lymphatic system, and blood system. Mature beet greens can be cooked; their young and tender versions can be added to salads. Carrot greens, too, are rich in nutrients, containing six times more vitamin C than the orange root, as well as potassium, calcium, and phytonutrients; these often-discarded parts can also add depth of flavor and complexity to dishes as an herb or side. Grape leaves have long been used in Mediterranean cultures for their anti-inflammatory properties, low glycemic load, and nutrient-rich profile. And the wolfberry leaves left over by the goji berry plant were my favorite sautéed greens during my travels in China.

A zero-waste study on the Korean radish, mu

The Korean radish, mu, is a variety of white radish with a firm, crunchy texture. Shorter and rounder than the Japanese daikon radish with a slightly green top, mu is favored in Korean cuisine for its denser texture and sweeter flavor. The whole mu, from its greens to its peel to its stem, can be eaten, and below I will show you how to use the whole plant approach using a single large radish. Mu also serves as an example of what we stand to gain when we try different kinds of vegetables than those that are typically used. The Korean radish, and radishes of all kinds, are packed with vitamins and nutrients: 5 times more vitamin C, 1½ times more iron, and 5 times more calcium than broccoli, and are known for glucosinolates, which scientists have linked to stimulating enzymes that deactivate carcinogens and decrease cancer cells' ability to spread.

The green leaves

Trim the greens from the top of each radish and wash them. Submerge them in a bowl of water with a splash of white vinegar to rinse off any dirt and sand. Wait a few minutes until the sediment sinks to the bottom of your bowl. Drain and repeat a few times. Then cook your radish greens by using the method of sigeumchi namul (spinach banchan); see page 48. Lightly cooking the greens, which mellows their peppery and pungent flavor, is a delicious way to enjoy them.

The outer peel

To make radish peel banchan, clean a radish with a vegetable scrubber to wash off dirt. Then use a vegetable peeler to remove the outer peel in thin strips. Heat a skillet over medium-high heat, and once the pan is hot, add 1 to 2 tablespoons of toasted sesame oil. Allow the oil to heat for 30 seconds, then add the peels and cook for 30 seconds. Remove the peels from the heat and dress with salt and sesame seeds to taste.

The flesh

In Korean cooking, the main body of the mu is used in its raw state, made into kimchi (like on page 22), or cooked. Raw, the main body can be freshly grated, resulting in something that looks a bit like snow. In its raw state, mu will contain living digestive enzymes that facilitate the digestion of proteins, carbohydrates, and fats. Koreans like to use the freshness of this unique grating of mu to pair with more oily dishes, like grilled mackerel. Or you can steam the flesh, cutting it into thin strips to top rice or serve as a side. It's delicious when you add a bit of soy sauce, toasted sesame oil, and gochugaru (red chili flakes).

The stem

After thoroughly cleaning the radish, I like to use the trimmed-off stems in hot pots or broth and stock recipes. Or you can compost them.

Royal Cuisine & Plant Diversity

"Biodiversity starts in the distant past, and it points to the future."

—*Frans Lanting,* **National Geographic** *photographer and environmental conservationist*

A Korean palace stands in Hanyang, what is now known as Seoul, a location that was well chosen to protect and feed its people. It is encircled by mountains and runs alongside the Cheonggyecheon Stream, which flows into an important trade route through the Han River. The location is also filled with a variety of rich landscapes that the plants draw nutrients and microbes from. Wild roots, herbs, and ferns are gathered from the mountainside; seaweed and algae are pulled from the seas; mushrooms and berries are foraged from the forests. These ingredients are brought by the locals to the palace as tributes to the king, each cherished for its natural properties to address ailments. In the palace kitchen, these gnarly plants are tamed of their wildness, dirt washed, skins scrubbed, and they are transformed into a fantastically elaborate royal cuisine.

Preparations for the king's meals start before sunrise when the royal kitchen begins to prepare one of five meals, which are under instructions from the palace physicians. Royal cuisine involved a close collaboration between the king's physicians and his cooks—a unique combination of flavor, the most current medicinal knowledge of the day, and decadent food presentation. In daily royal memos, the king's staff meticulously document his reactions to food, his symptoms, and any medical conditions he develops. If the king is ill, he is given a mixed herbal tea with ingredients targeted to treat his symptoms. Otherwise, his main course is an easily digestible porridge, fortified with pine nuts, ground apricot stone, jujubes, white and black sesame seeds, abalone, and mushrooms. On one side of the table is also a soup made of fermented shrimp, oysters, white radish, pollack roe, and zucchini. On the other, an assortment of

traditional banchan, small seasonal sides, such as kimchi, dried anchovies, seaweed, mussels, and sea cucumbers. His table is set with unique
bangjja, bronze tableware made with a 1:9 tin to copper ratio, ideal for
serving healthy food, for it retains heat better, can be sterilized, releases
minerals when water is stored in it, and even discolors when a trace of
pesticide, poison, or food with high sodium levels touches its surface.

At the palace, the concept of yak sik don gwon is in place: Food is
treated like precious medicine. This becomes a philosophy that trickles
down and is adopted by the people throughout the kingdom. The time-
honored wisdom of traditional food preparations—ferments, wine,
rice, and dooboo (tofu) making—fall under the jurisdiction of separate
official ministries, each with strict accountability for quality control.
The fermented sauces—the jangs and other condiments—are the
responsibility of the Royal Institute of Medicine and Pharmaceuticals.
Tending to the large outdoor vats of ferments for sauces and condiments
is arguably one of the most important tasks of the palace. The jars are
kept under lock and key, meticulously organized by fermentation age,
and require constant monitoring and adjustment.

In this way, every detail in these intricate food preparations is highly
considered to promote the health of the king. It is essential that the palace staff understand how key ingredients are grown in various local eco-
systems, as well as how food impacts the human body. To accumulate this
impressive body of knowledge, the palace staff spend most of their lives
within the palace walls, working to master the complex and ever-growing
body of knowledge of the diverse plants that make up the royal diet.

Plant diversity for modern life

The Joseon Dynasty, with it its elaborate royal cuisine, was the last of
its kind in Korea. For me, this slice of history serves as a fascinating

look into how yak sik dong won could be taken to its fullest form. I first heard about royal cuisine from the Buddhist nuns, who explained that palace cooks used to join the monasteries after retirement. My interest piqued, I began studying Korean royal cuisine and speaking with chefs specializing in it. I visited fine dining restaurants focused on re-creating royal cuisine, and I experienced what extreme plant diversity might have been like in the past. I tasted things like fresh napa cabbage pickled with matrimony vine, balloon flower, licorice, and lingzhi mushrooms, and sweetened with the natural flavors of chestnut honey and pear. I had soup made from dried pollack and ate rice bowls mixed with varied bracken sprouts, and served with aged beef. I imagined my ancestors walking through uncut meadows and forests to find and gather these ingredients.

My busy, modern lifestyle had made eating in the traditional way difficult. I relied on conveniences like restaurants, takeout, and packaged foods when I didn't make the time or have the interest to cook. However, as I learned more about royal cuisine and the mechanics of how these meals were constructed, I was inspired to discover that many of the dishes I had grown up with were founded on these very concepts. Was there a way to translate a more simplified version, with the same health benefits, for my daily routine? Then the answer came to me: I could re-create the diverse plant experience of royal cuisine by making simple, assorted banchan with the jangs at breakfast, lunch, and dinner. To make things even easier, I would forgo the little bowls traditionally used to serve banchan and put them all on the same plate or in a bowl (see Elements of a Longevity Meal on page 100). And at the end of each week, or whenever I needed to clear my refrigerator, I would incorporate leftovers, something I saw the Buddhist nuns do. My favorite practice now is to use leftover ingredients to creatively assemble a new dish.

Kimchi bokkeumbap (kimchi pan-fried rice)

Kimchi pan-fried rice, also known as kimchi bokkeumbap, is a classic comfort food in Korean cuisine. It is made by lightly stir-frying kimchi and rice, along with seasonings and really any topping that you like. The versatility of this dish allows me to use up leftovers in the refrigerator in a way that is tasty and wholesome, even as a side dish. You can similarly use up leftovers when cooking other dishes too, like in curries and stir-fries.

INGREDIENTS

Serves 4

1½ teaspoons olive oil

½ teaspoon minced garlic

½ cup meat, cooked or raw (steak, beef, chicken, bacon), minced

1 cup kimchi, plus the juice, which is found at the bottom of the kimchi container

½ cup leftover produce from the refrigerator (mushrooms, spinach, ssukgat, bean sprouts), minced

3 cups steamed rice

1½ teaspoons toasted sesame oil

4 large eggs, cooked sunny-side up or scrambled

Sesame seeds, chopped green onion, and/or roasted seaweed strips, for garnish (optional)

METHOD

1. Set a wide, flat pan or skillet over medium-high heat and add the olive oil and garlic. Cook, stirring, until fragrant, about 1 minute.

2. If you have any uncooked meat, add it now and cook for a few minutes, until half-cooked. Otherwise, add the kimchi and cook for 2 minutes, followed by the leftover meat, leftover produce, kimchi juice, and rice. Continue to cook this for about 7 minutes, then take the pan off the heat. Add the sesame oil as a finishing touch and mix well.

3. Divide the rice among bowls. Garnish with cooked eggs, sesame seeds, green onion, and/or seaweed strips, if using.

4. Eat immediately or store in the refrigerator in an airtight container for up to 5 to 7 days.

Everyday greens: sigeumchi namul (spinach banchan)

Sigeumchi namul, seasoned spinach, is perhaps the most popular Korean banchan side dish. You can also swap the spinach in this recipe for other vegetables, like ssukgat, watercress, or kale. Cooking namul is a great way to explore what's in season and to extend the life of leftover ingredients in your fridge. The key here is the recipe's quick boiling cooking method—blanching—which removes the bitter taste of the wild greens while retaining as much of the plant's nutrients as possible. In my research, I found it fascinating that long-lived populations in Greece use a similar basic greens recipe daily—horta, boiled wild leafy greens, splashed with olive oil and lemon.

Recipe notes

Gukganjang is a special traditionally brewed soy sauce made as a by-product of making doenjang (Korean fermented beans), which adds an umami flavor. It can be found on Amazon or at a specialty Asian grocer.

Heat breaks down plant cell walls, making cooked greens easier to digest than raw, but the heat also denatures the plant, bringing down its nutrients. By blanching your greens, you expose them to as little heat as possible.

INGREDIENTS

Serves 2, as a side

1 bunch spinach

1 teaspoon minced garlic

1½ teaspoons gukganjang (Korean soup soy sauce) or ¾ teaspoon other naturally brewed soy sauce

1 teaspoon toasted sesame oil

1 teaspoon sesame seeds (optional)

2 to 3 teaspoons gochujang (red pepper paste), or a sprinkle of gochugaru (red chili flakes), for added spice (optional)

METHOD

1. Prepare a medium bowl of ice water.

2. In a medium pot, bring 2 cups filtered water to a boil over high heat. Add the spinach and blanch for 20 seconds, or until wilted. Quickly remove the spinach from the boiling water and immerse in the prepared bowl of ice water to stop the cooking process. Drain the spinach and gently squeeze out excess water.

3. Put the spinach in a bowl and add the garlic, soy sauce, sesame oil, and, if using, sesame seeds and gochujang or gochugaru. Mix by hand until well combined, then cut the spinach into 2-inch pieces.

4. Serve immediately or refrigerate in an airtight container for up to 3 days.

Everyday banchan and namul

Royal cooks during the Joseon period relied on banchan to anchor every meal. These banchan included small plant-based dishes called namul, made from the mushrooms, roots, and wild greens surrounding the palace. The healthy cooking methods used in these dishes were key to nutrient absorption and digestion. Ingredients were fermented, or they were gently cooked, then seasoned with a bit of toasted sesame oil, salt, or soy sauce.

In Korean culture, banchan is served every day, whether you are having a simple meal at home or celebrating a holiday like Chuseok, Korean Thanksgiving Day. Banchan is meant to be a side dish, to complement a main meal, bringing a unique richness with every bite. But banchan can be enjoyed as meals in and of themselves, with just a bit of rice if you like. Banchan dishes are a delightful surprise for anyone just discovering Korean cuisine. They are also a flavorful solution to tame the natural bitterness of the most nutrient-dense plants, the bitter flavor that has been shown to aid digestion, help nutrient absorption, stimulate immune function, and even help curb sugar cravings.

Korean ssam, using perilla leaves

The royal palace also served ssam, which involved plucking the freshest seasonal leaves, like lettuce and perilla leaves, from the palace garden. Fermented bean or chile paste, rice, and a mix of any of the ingredients offered at the table were tucked into the raw leaves, essentially used as wrappers, for a delightful mouth explosion with every bite.

For me, this is a delicious and versatile way to increase the plant diversity in your meals and use leftovers in the refrigerator. The basic ingredient is gochujang (red pepper paste) and a green leaf. As long as you have these base ingredients, your ssam ingredients are really up to your imagination. You can add rice, grilled meat, kimchi, gochujang, garlic, jalapeño, banchan, or other cooked vegetables.

Place the perilla leaf flat on your hand, or do what I call the double ssam method and add an additional layer of red or other leafy lettuce. Fold the leaves to tuck in the ingredients. (This does not have to be precise.) Enjoy the ssam like a mini sandwich or wrap.

Mighty phytochemicals and the power of plant color

The Joseon palace kitchen knew then what science has now confirmed: Eating a broad and rotating plant base matters for our health. The reasons are twofold: The first is because of the benefits of plant diversity to our gut flora, and the second is the health benefits we reap through nutrient-rich phytochemicals found in plants.

Phytochemicals, first described in the 1950s by American biochemist Julius Axelrod, are still a relatively new concept in the health world. Since no single food contains all of our required nutrients, we must eat a wide variety of foods to ensure that we get all of our essential nutrients. These nutrients traditionally include protein, carbohydrates, and E, B, A, C, and K vitamins. But emerging research includes a new essential category: phytochemicals, which are bioactive nutrient chemicals found in plants.

Scientists currently estimate there are more than ten thousand phytochemicals, which are still being explored to define their full impact on human health. The most studied phytochemicals are those that have **antioxidant** (anti-aging) power, compounds that give plants their different tastes, smells, and richly colored rainbow hues as well as white, brown, and black plant colors that are extremely important in Asian cuisine for medicinal value. Antioxidant phytochemicals fall into two major groups: **carotenoids**, exhibiting bright orange, red, and yellow hues found in tomatoes, carrots, and mangoes; and **polyphenols,** which include flavonoids, found in berries, citrus, onions, soybeans, and coffee. Recent studies have also linked **sulfur-rich** compounds to be significant for human health; these are found in cabbage (think kimchi), onions, and mushrooms, foods that have had a long medicinal history in Asian cuisine.

Phytochemicals are an exciting new frontier in functional foods, offering health benefits beyond meeting basic nutrition needs. With a better understanding of these bioactive compounds, we can move toward a more systematic approach to identifying them on nutrient labels and utilizing our ancestral wisdom in plant medicines derived from our natural environments. There is evidence to suggest that phytochemicals can help us build resistance to every known chronic disease—cancer, heart disease, diabetes, autoimmune diseases, the list goes on—as well as benefiting every part of our bodies, from our brain to our eyes, skin, hair, and joints. Emerging research reveals enormous potential for the use of phytochemicals to improve our health. One can imagine a future where standardized phytochemical bioactivity numbers are located prominently on nutrition labels, information currently missing, to help consumers make more informed purchasing choices.

Since 2012, the American Gut Project has collected crowdsourced bacterial samples from more than eleven thousand individuals living in forty-five countries across the globe. To date, these samples reveal that individuals whose weekly diet includes more than thirty different types of plants had some correspondence with reduced inflammation and cardiovascular disease.[1] Plant diversity helps our bodies to function at their best.

Scientific evidence also shows that we benefit from eating the living enzymes found in raw (or uncooked) plants, better still if healthy bacteria from the living fertile soil it was grown in is embedded in the produce (i.e., it matters where your produce comes from). However, eating a 100 percent raw diet is not easy on the digestive system and not ideal for most people, as it can result in bloating and difficulty absorbing nutrients, particularly for those with underlying health conditions. The best nutritional approach for most of us is to eat both raw and cooked vegetables and to choose mostly gentle cooking methods in order to retain the plant's nutritional profile and digestive enzymes.

Beyond broccoli: The benefits of eating golgoru

Eating golgoru in Korea means eating with balance, plant diversity, and variety, without leaving anything behind and discouraging food waste. The notion drives how meals are put together in a traditional Korean setting and how eating many kinds of things is encouraged.

According to the food company Green Giant, in 2022, broccoli was America's favorite vegetable, bypassing the once beloved potato. Broccoli is hailed as one of the healthiest vegetables, with high fiber and high vitamin C and K content, along with a range of other nutrients. No doubt, broccoli is a vegetable that should be ubiquitously considered in daily diets, as it is easily accessible, low in calories, and nutrient dense. But what if we pushed ourselves to consider other ways to use delicious, nutritious plants that are less commonly known and hidden in plain sight?

Two plants from traditional Korean cuisine—persimmons and perilla leaves—provide illuminating examples of what can happen when we expand our palates. Often used in ssam, perilla leaves, as well as smaller, daintier Japanese shiso leaves, contain thirteen times more vitamin A, nine times more manganese (for bone health), six times more calcium, four times more vitamin K, and almost double the fiber when compared to broccoli.[2] Perilla leaves are a favorite in my household, and we eat them in a variety of different ways, sharing a stack of the raw leaves to make ssam, cutting them up in bits as a fresh herb topper, or using them in sandwiches. They are delicious, adding texture and minty flavor to dishes, whether chopped up, used in ssam wraps, or ground into nourishing broths. While perilla leaves are typically found in specialty Asian groceries, you can utilize the ssam technique to experiment and rotate any seasonal leafy variety at your local store, like red lettuce leaves, dinosaur kale, steamed or raw cabbage leaves, red chicory leaves, or bok choy leaves. Really, it's up to your imagination.

Persimmon, the Asian cousin to the apple, offers forty-seven times more vitamin C, ninety-eight times more vitamin A, and more potassium, calcium, folate, and fiber than the apple.[3] Persimmons come in both crunchy versions (which taste like milder, cinnamon-flavored apples) and soft versions (with more of a cinnamon-mango flavor). They are featured prominently in Korean and Japanese cuisines, as a unique dried fruit snack, or as a natural sweetener added to prepared dishes and even to spicy kimchi.

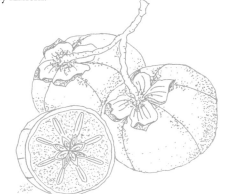

When we think beyond what is on the standard plate, we can find ways to maximize our health while also trying new foods that are exciting and delicious. As I began to learn about the various plants within my heritage and their natural properties, they became delightful new additions to my meals: a fistful of newly discovered fresh greens that would crown my stews or be nestled as banchan within my increasingly colorful plate. I knew each mouthful would make me stronger and healthier. Celery varieties, for example, are often used in Asian cuisine and juiced, raw, or lightly cooked offer a budget-friendly antidote to bloating and inflammation.

Ssukgat, another powerful example, is believed to be a detoxifying agent and used as a diuretic; it is also used for heart health, to protect the body against colds, to curb sugar cravings, to improve skin and hair health, and to prevent kidney stones, bloating, and bone loss. In Asia, it is known as "cold medicine you can eat." Ssukgat is a nod to all of the other highly nutritious Asian greens often featured in Korean royal court cuisine. Much like minari, which in Lee Isaac Chung's 2020 film of the same name is described as eaten by beggars and millionaires, ssukgat symbolizes self-care that is accessible to all, especially when we eat golgoru.

Plant diversity benefits the planet

In 1831, twenty-two-year-old Charles Darwin took the trip of a lifetime, invited aboard the HMS *Beagle* for a five-year journey as the ship's naturalist to study and take field notes on exotic plants and animals. He brought with him no advanced tools, just notebooks and pencils, and traversed the world—to the coasts of Africa, South America, and the Galápagos Islands—exploring, documenting, and collecting thousands of unknown species. Darwin's experience ultimately led him

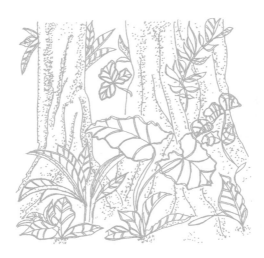

to pen the famous *On the Origin of Species*, which included a simple sketched tree diagram to illustrate his theory of evolution, a theory that would radically change our understanding of the natural world.

Today, although we have high-tech equipment, evidence-based studies, and photographers staffed to record the extreme reaches of our planet, we still haven't been able to create an accurate library of the world's plant diversity. Nor have we been able to prove through definitive scientific studies exactly how specific plants can help optimize our health. Part of the gap in our understanding lies in the fact that we still do not have a full picture of all the plant-based resources available to us on our planet.

It would seem beneficial to our existence to close this knowledge gap, as it is estimated that a whopping 80 percent of Earth's biomass is composed of plants, with bacteria coming in second at 13 percent, and fungus coming in third at 2 percent. In comparison, we humans are barely a rounding error, making up just 0.01 percent of this composition. The United Nations Food and Agriculture Organization counts

300,000 plant species that are currently known to be edible. However, just three of these plant species—rice, corn, and wheat—contribute to almost 60 percent of the Western diet. This means that not only is there still much to be discovered in our plant-based world, but also that we are not using much of what we do know. In the past, scientists like Darwin and the residents of ancient Korean kingdoms sought to close this gap in plant knowledge simply by exploring and observing. We can try to do the same, even with small, everyday tasks like grocery shopping.

How I became a zero-waste grocery forager

Once I committed to eating with more plant diversity, I started planning my meals and shopping for groceries differently. I imagined how my ancestors might have foraged for the season's best ingredients. I also began to think about how I would go zero waste with food.

First, I check to see what I already have on hand to avoid doubles. I plan how to eat what would spoil first. To save time, I list my grocery items according to how they appear in my favorite local market. Then, once I'm at the market, I think like a grocery forager, exploring the diversity I encounter. I like to take a cue from Charles Darwin and use simple powers of observation to make purchasing choices on what will come freshest to me at the market. Is it in season with maximum nutrients or imported with nutrients lost during transportation miles? I focus on procuring whole foods and natural ingredients, reducing packed and processed foods, leaving them naked in my shopping basket without plastic bags as much as possible.

When I get home, I store my ingredients to make them last longer. I extend the life of herbs, stemmed produce (e.g., asparagus), and root vegetables (e.g., carrots and celery) by treating them like plants. I remove rubber bands and ties, trim the bottom of their stems, store them submerged in water, and change the water every four to five days or when the water gets cloudy. This way, I can keep my asparagus and celery healthy for up to two weeks and my carrots for up to one month.

Thinking like a zero-waste forager has made grocery shopping a lot more fun. I get creative with leftovers and really don't mind deviating from my list if I see something that piques my curiosity, all in the name of exploring the planet's plant diversity.

Plant diversity for the time-pressed

Few of us live in royal palaces with a kitchen staff at our disposal to gather ingredients or in monasteries where we have the time to slowly ferment our foods and prepare our meals. It might seem like a challenge to increase the plant diversity in our diets, but it can be easier than we think. When I walk through GrowNYC's Union Square Greenmarket in Manhattan, I note that even in an urban setting, fresh, organic ingredients are readily accessible if we know where to look for them.

Remember the Buddhist nuns' discreet lazy Susan filled with medicinal condiments, including fermented pastes? What about the king's meals filled with small side dishes and soups simmered with healthful ingredient mixtures? Often overlooked, these foundational sides and ingredients offer powerful diversity in nutrients and antioxidant phytochemicals, and they make it easy to significantly boost the nutrient density in our diets and aid digestion for maximum nutrient absorption.

Here are a few easy and fun ways to emulate the nuns' and kings' approach, updated for the current century.

- Curate your own healthy condiments tray or lazy Susan—you can make your own tray of extra condiments at the table, like Korean gochujang, soy sauce, and black vinegar

- Easy, everyday banchan—at the start of each week, you can prepare batches of simple banchan or other simply prepared produce, like roasted vegetables, to store in your fridge for healthy sides to cover plant diversity
- Final layers—sprinkle or splash raw plant-based ingredients like citrus juice, spices (e.g., pepper, cinnamon), dried powders (e.g., algae, mushroom), or fresh herbs (e.g., scallions, thyme)
- Explore the canned or frozen section—like canned water chestnuts and beans or frozen peas for ready additions in your kitchen
- Add plant-diverse dishes—including soups, broth, and stir-fries
- Cook noodles with leftover greens and other vegetables

When you are rushed and maximizing plant diversity in your diet is a challenge, consider Canada's food guide, which recommends at least one dark green and one bright orange (or red or yellow) vegetable or fruit per day. Green and orange tend to be the brighter hues that are easiest to find in the markets, in the form of vegetables like carrots, broccoli, or tomatoes, and they come with an incredible range of nutritional benefits. Orange hues provide powerful antioxidants—lycopene and beta-carotenes—and are rich in vitamin A, vitamin C, potassium, and fiber; green hues also have beta-carotenes, omega-3s and another powerful antioxidant, glucoraphanin, and are rich in vitamin A, potassium, calcium, folate, and fiber. I personally take this a step further, aiming to always have a different dark green vegetable at every meal. Dark green vegetables, especially Asian greens such as ssukgat, perilla leaves, pea shoots, and bok choy, pack a nutritional punch with their high levels of fiber, iron, magnesium, potassium, calcium, and folate.

Jeongol (Korean-style hot pot)

Hot pot holds a regular spot on our family menu because it naturally lends to family time, not to mention a delicious way to get plant diversity in. Hot pot has a long history in Asian culture, dating back to dynasty cooking in royal kitchens, and was used for centuries to stretch available ingredients in a flavorful way. The more simplified versions were stews, or Korean jjigaes. It's the ultimate expression of communal bonding, with friends and family gathering over a steaming pot filled with flavorful broth and loads of vegetables they get to cook together. I have adapted this recipe to accommodate an ever-changing plant-diverse meal. Here, I have laid out many variations on broth and ingredient choice for hot pot across Asia. You can build your hot pot by choosing your preference of ingredients from each of the following categories: broth, noodle or rice, vegetables, protein, and sauces/other toppings. Feel free to swap in similar ingredients, using whatever you have in the refrigerator.

INGREDIENTS

Serves 4

4 cups broth of choice (like the anchovy broth on page 116, chicken, etc.) or water

6 to 8 ounces choice of noodles (like rice, potato, kelp) or 3 to 4 cups cooked rice

3 to 4 ounces leafy greens (like white cabbage, ssukgat, leeks, bok choy, lettuce)

METHOD

1. Pour the broth into a large pot. Arrange the noodles, leafy greens, mushrooms, root vegetables, and protein in the pot, bring to a boil over high heat, then lower the heat. Cover with a lid and simmer until your protein of choice is cooked through, about 5 minutes. Serve family style, alongside personal bowls of dipping sauce and other toppings.

1 to 2 (8-ounce) packets mushrooms (like enoki, oyster, black wood ear)

2 to 4 ounces root vegetables (like Korean radish, carrots, lotus roots, bamboo shoots)

1 to 2 pounds protein (like sliced tofu, thinly sliced beef, thinly sliced raw red snapper, deveined shrimp, fish balls)

Your choice of dipping sauce and other toppings, including:

Gluten-free raw tahini (or traditional sesame paste)

Gluten-free coconut aminos (or soy sauce), vinegar, crushed chili, and coriander

Gluten-free coconut aminos (or soy sauce) mixed with squeeze of lemon juice, mirin, and bonito flakes

Raw egg yolk

Chili oil

Minced fresh garlic

Chopped fresh cilantro

Chopped scallions

Kimchi

2. Alternatively, you can blanch your choice of ingredients at the dining table using an electric hot pot burner or portable heat source. Place your pot on the heat source set in the middle of the dining table. Arrange the selection of your ingredients in small dishes surrounding the pot. Seat your fellow diners around the hot pot and encourage them to use communal chopsticks and a ladle to portion out ingredients and broth into personal bowls.

3. Allow each person to blanch their desired ingredients by picking up ingredients with communal chopsticks, stirring the ingredients in the broth for a few seconds, and transferring to their personal bowl of dipping sauce. Start with tough vegetables and tofu first, then softer vegetables. Sturdier root vegetables take longer to cook; thin meat slices take only a few seconds.

Still, too much of one specific plant can lead to toxin build-up in our bodies (because each plant naturally contains a small amount of toxin to protect it from predators). Therefore, a rotation and variety in the plants that we eat is key.

Feeding the next generation

The more I learned about plant diversity, the more curious I became. Every time I encountered a new ingredient, I would do a deep dive on its nutritional profile, either on PubMed (pubmed.ncbi.nlm.nih.gov), which freely shares scientific articles to the public and is maintained by the National Center for Biotechnology Information (NCBI) at the National Institutes of Health (NIH), or on a nutrient tracking site like FoodData Central (fdc.nal.usda.gov/fdc-app.html#/), which is published by the US Department of Agriculture. Researching was helpful for me to understand the benefits of these new-to-me ingredients. This exploration greatly expanded my repertoire beyond the usual suspects like broccoli, kale, spinach, and cauliflower.

It was an adventure, especially in Asia, where I found many of the ingredients were wobbly and imperfect, different from the pristine produce that I was used to from my Americanized upbringing. In the process of opening my mind to this whole new world of plant-based edibles, I dispelled any previous notions of what I considered to be too "exotic" or "strange" and started appreciating and respecting what different cultures had been enjoying as food throughout the globe.

I also tried many things to get my kids to eat more vegetables. I initially hid their vegetables in sauces and soups, but I realized that this wouldn't improve their real food literacy. I switched to making things taste better and rotating and experimenting until, through trial and error, I found plant-based dishes they liked. I rotated simple seasonal produce plates, introducing new items for them to choose at breakfast. I roasted vegetables with a sprinkle of salt to help with the natural bitterness of greens, and I lightly stir-fried bacon in vegetables with a squeeze of lemon to add a flavor twist. The trickiest part was finding plant-based dishes that they were willing to eat for breakfast, as I believe in the importance of getting critical nutrients at the start of the day to provide us with a foundation of energy and a metabolism boost.

My solution became to prepare a quick, nutrient-dense seasonal breakfast platter of greens and fruits that includes both raw and lightly cooked vegetables, low-glycemic fruits, and small amounts of dried sea-weed sheets, served family-style and placed at the center of our dining table. This way, because we all wake up and eat at different times, we can take what we want as we please. I make sure to prepare a rotating mix of items so that, over time, we are ingesting a varied supply of healthy bacteria and active digestive enzymes. The point is that you are taking in some variety of produce, mostly greens, to start your day. The platter can be as simple or as varied as you want in the morning. I like to use gentle cooking methods because they limit the time at the heat source, which can degenerate nutrient levels, to keep the enzymes alive (some-where between 110 and 120°F). Preparing this platter is usually very quick, especially if some are ingredients left over from dinner the night before.

Just as I had rethought breakfast, I did the same for all our meals. I dropped any previous notions about what they should look like, thinking instead about how I could add nutrients that our family had not eaten in the previous meal, for even more layers of plant diversity and nutrients over the day. For example, if I had blanched ssukgat in the morning, then I would choose other vegetables for the rest of our meals, like endive for my lunch salad or lightly cooked carrots for din-ner. In this framework of varying my plant nutrients as much as possible within a single day, I ignored typical mealtime labels for foods—for example, eating shakshuka, the Middle Eastern stewed tomato-egg dish usually eaten for breakfast, for lunch or dinner. And I tried to think like a forager, introducing edible plants from different environments and elevation points—like mushrooms from the forest, algae from the sea, and turmeric or cabbage from the land—into our daily diet in order to benefit our microbiota.

As we started focusing on real food and an increased level of plant diversity, everyone in the household started to transform in their own way. While I was getting stronger day by day with more bounce to my steps, I noticed a new rosy glow in my kids' cheeks. At the same time, they were growing remarkably taller, shooting up like little plants. My son, an avid meat lover, had previously declared that he would no longer eat vegetables. But along this journey, he became a student athlete and decided that plant-based ingredients would be a core part of his fitness regimen. For my math whiz kid who started reading at eighteen months old, I needed to apply logic to his young brain to convince him to change his mind. He needed to understand the whys and see the research. I was tickled when he told me one day, "Mama, if you don't eat vegetables, you'll get sick." Even my daughter, who had already seen the benefits of and enjoyed produce, shot up from her tiny frame when we added more nutrient-rich plants to the mix. And, to my delight, she began to self-study, going deeper into Korean culture and language. I began to notice Hangul, the Korean alphabet, feverishly scribbled in her notebooks at night. Growing up in Hong Kong, my kids learned Mandarin. But my daughter was pushing herself to read and write in the language of her second identity. Wherever she goes, she is thrilled every time she can read and understand Korean.

SUN

Ssukgat thrives with sunlight. Beneath the warmth of the sun's rays, this plant will flourish and bloom, sharing its gifts year-round. At the same time, if left for hours without shade on long summer days, ssukgat can wither. The sun is so powerful, we need to respect its strength and use it in moderation.

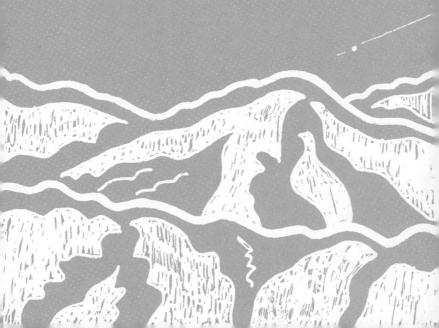

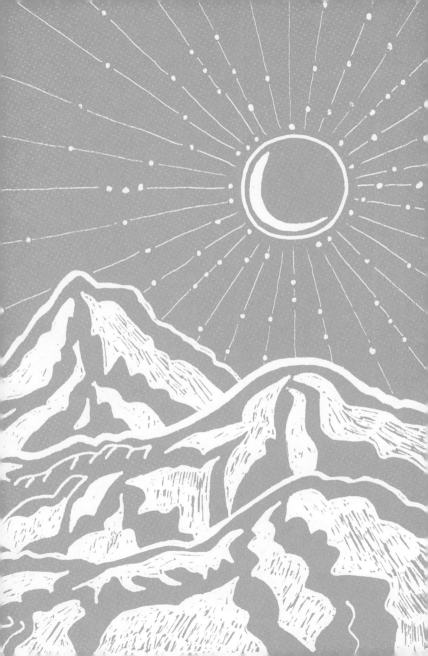

Sunshine, Fresh Air & Dirt

"The six best doctors in the world, and no one can deny it, are sunshine, water, rest, and air, exercise and diet. These six will gladly you attend, if only you are willing. Your mind they'll ease, your will they'll mend, and charge you not one shilling."[1]

—*Wayne Fields, memoirist,* **What the River Knows**

I distinctly remember a day years ago when I was working in a looming skyscraper in New York City, from an office with lots of walled cubicles and fluorescent lights. In front of the building was a small patch of grass with a few benches arranged neatly. On this day, the weather was balmy and lovely. I could hear birds chirping in the one tree we had on the lawn. My teammates and I had lined up to buy our midday meal from the regular food truck that parked outside with our favorite coffee and bagels.

Waiting for my turn, I watched as a senior executive finished the tuna and veggie wrap he had brought from home before proceeding to lie flat on the grass—suit and all—and fall into a deep sleep. We all laughed and nudged each other. He had probably just finished working an all-nighter, which was a common occurrence for all of us. But my colleague had been wise to pack a healthy lunch and eat it under the warmth of that cloudless sky—perhaps the one chance he would get that day before heading back indoors to work until evening. I marched back inside, without another thought, to eat my food truck lunch at my desk. Looking back, though, I realize he was on to something.

The sunshine vitamin

Some fascinating recent discoveries have been made about the importance of vitamin D and exposure to bacteria through soil and air to our immune system and microbiome. These discoveries disprove previous recommendations telling us to avoid the sun and hyper-sterilize our environments.

We know that vitamin D is essential for building and maintaining healthy bones and for reducing our risk of disease. Research has shown that high levels of vitamin D reduce the risk of multiple sclerosis, inflammatory bowel diseases, and osteoporosis. There is also promising new research that suggests a link between vitamin D and disease prevention for type 1 diabetes and COVID-19. However, most of the modern world's population is not getting enough vitamin D.

In a cross-hospital study done in Vancouver, scientists set out to study the connection between gut microbiota, vitamin D, and exposure to sunlight.[2] They found that exposing research participants to ultraviolet B light (UVB) over one week increased vitamin D production by 10 percent. Additionally, participants' vitamin D levels increased their microbiome diversity and, with it, their immunity. The researchers concluded that vitamin D and sunlight are critical for gut microbiome health and immune function.

When we don't get enough vitamin D, we can experience fatigue, bone/joint/muscle pain, more frequent illness, anxiety, weight gain, and hair loss. There are dietary sources of vitamin D, but it may be difficult for the average individual to eat enough vitamin-D-rich foods daily to get their levels to where they should be. The easiest way to get enough vitamin D is through regular exposure to sunlight. For most of us, spending ten to fifteen minutes outside in the sun with our arms and legs exposed is all that is required—dependent, of course, on where we live. If you live in a climate where year-round sun exposure is not possible (or if you have an underlying health condition that affects vitamin D production), you should ask your doctor to test your vitamin D levels to see if supplementation is required beyond diet and regular sunlight exposure. And, of course, when you do spend time in the sun, make sure to protect your skin from too much sun, which is associated with skin cancers and sunburn.

Beyond vitamin D, allowing sunlight to enter your eye retina at the beginning of the day, and obtaining as much natural daylight throughout the day, also serves the critical function of helping your body to build up melatonin, a chemical in your brain that helps you to regulate your body's internal clock to get optimal sleep. There is also research that sun exposure increases serotonin levels, which help to regulate mood and make us less prone to anxiety and depression.

If you spend a lot of time working inside an office or on a computer, it is essential to find ways to get more natural sunlight into your system, perhaps during your lunch break. This is an easy lifestyle shift that can greatly impact your health. When I wake up in the morning, I make sure that sunlight hits my eyes to set my internal clock for the day by opening my windows first thing in the morning. Then, throughout the day, I try to sensibly expose myself to sunlight—by walking, hiking, playing sports, or sitting outside in the park. I never knew that feeling the warm sun on my skin could feel this good.

The value of getting dirty

A growing body of scientific research supports the health benefits of spending more time outdoors and living in harmony with the natural elements as our ancestors did. These recent discoveries support what my former colleague was doing by napping in the sun. Scientists have not only made discoveries about the importance of sunlight, they now also understand that exposure to bacteria, through soil and air, improves our health.

As the Buddhist nuns and the ancient kings knew, beneficial bacteria help us to build a healthy microbiome and boost our immune system. But even if your microbiome has been depleted—due to health issues or a poor diet—Dr. Robynne Chutkan, an integrative gastroenterologist and author of *The Microbiome Solution*[3] believes "rewilding" the microbiome is possible through a clean diet that includes probiotics and "living a little dirtier" through exposure to rich, chemical-free soil, another one of nature's essential elements. Soil and air within forested areas contain millions of bacteria that contribute to the development of a healthy immune system. By interacting with the dirt and germs in these natural environments, as the Buddhist nuns and centenarians do, we are training our immune systems to respond appropriately in healthy ways. These natural environments also benefit our cardiovascular and metabolic systems by encouraging healthy bacteria, which fight against toxins, parasites, and pathogens, to grow and flourish.

Forest bathing is a popular activity, especially in Korea, for all ages, and is also used for its therapeutic effects. It is the simple practice of walking into the forest, taking in nature and the forest atmosphere around you while breathing deeply, all of which helps with rewilding, boosting immunity, de-stressing, and lifting your mood. So, forest bathe like the Koreans do by spending time in forests or near trees to increase your exposure to healthy microbiota from the soil and plants around you while reducing your stress hormone production by being close to nature. Or you can start to eat more fresh produce grown in rich, chemical-free soil to increase your exposure to good bacteria in the natural world around you.

It is estimated that the average person spends most of their time indoors due to modern lifestyles that revolve around driving, screen time, and work; take 93 percent of Americans, for example. As a result, we are exposed to very little microbial diversity. We have also become increasingly disconnected from the natural world around us. It's important to recognize that exposure to fresh air, sunlight, and soil not only benefits your microbiome but is good for your soul. Opportunities to be outside are omnipresent and free, even within the confines of city living.

Time spent outdoors is a surprisingly overlooked resource for preventative care and a healthy lifestyle.

Reconnecting with the natural world in Korea

Korea seamlessly and beautifully blends nature with urban life, as do other cities across the world, like Hong Kong and New York. Away from the blare of cars honking in traffic jams or people hurriedly walking on densely packed sidewalks, in Korea, I found peace and quiet whenever I got closer to nature there, be it along a scenic walkway of trees next to running water or smelling the fresh produce of greenmarkets.

Thoughtful urban planning in Seoul has facilitated healthy living for its citizens, allowing them easy access to sunshine and the outdoors amid a major urban center. Projects like the revitalization of Cheonggyecheon, which revived the historically important stream covered by concrete, and Seoul Skygarden, a new elevated park skyway, have transformed urban spaces to bring man-made parks and nature closer to city residents. In addition, a series of widespread changes were implemented to encourage residents to explore and bring nature intentionally into the city: widening sidewalks at the expense of car lanes, turning a large traffic circle into a circular green park, instituting a public bike share program, installing red clay paths for barefoot walking, reorganizing bus lines, and improving and expanding the already world-class train system. While you don't have to live in Seoul to connect with nature, you can experience outdoor time by walking, biking, or using public transportation to get around.

These were some of my favorite places in Korea to reconnect with the natural world.

Cheonggyecheon Stream

Walking along the Cheonggyecheon Stream* transported me back centuries when kings ruled during the Joseon Dynasty. In 2003, then-Seoul mayor Lee Myung-bak initiated a massive restoration, transforming the former highway previously covering the stream into a spectacular eco-friendly public park that reintroduced nature to the city, akin to NYC's High Line. For seven miles, I walked along the stream from east to west through downtown Seoul, listening to the rustling of tall grasses and the rush of waterfalls. I delighted in the elegant heron birds perched among the trees and sat on stepping stones inside the stream. At night, I saw gorgeous historical art and culture installations light up under the stars. Open twenty-four hours, it is a perfect place to bring friends and family or to spend time alone to see nature and its seasonal changes all year long. If I lived in Seoul, that's where I would be every day.

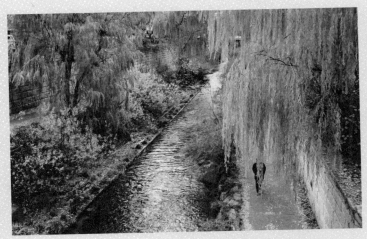

WALK NEAR NATURE AND OPEN WATER
TO RESTORE WELL-BEING

* Formerly known as the Gaecheon Stream during the Joseon Dynasty.

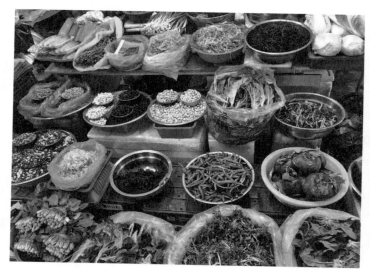

FIND NATURE'S BOUNTY IN A
TRADITIONAL STREET FOOD MARKET

Gwangjang Market

To see Korea's natural bounty all in one place, I visited the traditional street market, Gwangjang Market, at the end of the Cheonggyecheon Stream. This 42,000-square-foot space has 65,000 visitors each day. There was a fantastic array of hundreds of kimchi varieties, seaweeds, bracken, beans, and spices, as far as the eye can see. I sat down to try Korea's traditional foods, like jeon (savory pancakes), kimbap seaweed vegetable and rice wraps, and noodles made by the merchants in the market and imagined where on the land each of these foods must have blossomed before being picked to sell.

Crochet Trees

From fall to winter throughout Seoul, hundreds of trees are clothed in creative crocheted sweaters and blankets. Featuring hearts, flowers, and winter themes, the blankets help the trees live longer, as they are an effective measure against pests who enter the tree trunks for warmth during the winters. I found this act of clothing the trees to be a thoughtful gesture, taking care the environment while helping to encourage city dwellers to stroll by and reconnect with nature. A popular place to view them is Jeongdong-gil, a picturesque street where you can watch the trees change through the different stages of fall foliage. It is located within the Deoksugung Stonewall Walkway.

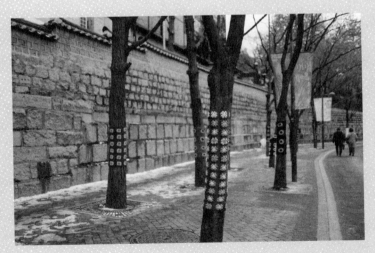

TAKE CARE OF THE ENVIRONMENT

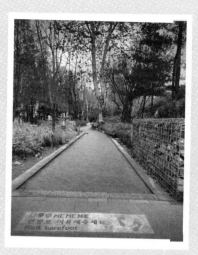

CONNECT YOUR BARE SKIN
WITH THE EARTH

Barefoot Paths

I had heard about red clay barefoot paths throughout Korea and visited one in Neulbeot Park, right in the middle of Seoul. Many Koreans believe in the importance of reconnecting with nature through barefoot walking, also known as "earthing" or "grounding," which has reported effects on chronic pain and muscle damage, as certain parts of the feet are connected to specific body parts. The Earth's surface contains free electrons that can be transferred to the human body upon direct contact, and these electrons then act as antioxidants to help neutralize free radicals in our bodies to reduce inflammation. There is a station where you can wash your feet after the walk.

Naejangsan National Park

I visited Naejangsan National Park to drink in the forest air, see the Buddhist nuns, and experience temple food. Forest bathing is a popular activity in Korea for all generations and has reported benefits, including improving cardiovascular function and immunity, reducing inflammation, and lowering blood pressure, heart rate, and levels of harmful hormones like cortisol, which your body produces when stressed.

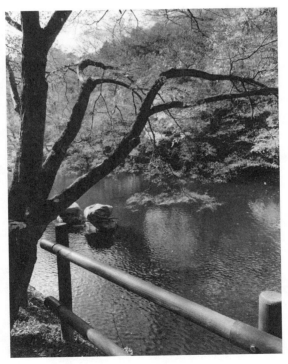

DRINK IN
THE FOREST AIR

Jeju Island

Jeju Island has been called the Hawaii of Korea and is beloved for its natural beauty. I felt like I had slipped back into a previous century when I saw the untouched natural landscapes of molten rock and visited the haenyeo, the female divers who live here and maintain the traditional practice of sea diving without breathing equipment. I highly recommend seeing the island's waterfalls, natural volcanic rock formations, and beautiful beaches, or trying the island's sweet Halla-bong tangerines. There is also the seven-mile Seogwipo Healing Forest to visit, with healing that comes with forest bathing, breathing in the clean air, and contemplating amid the quiet of its cypress and cedar trees. You can also try the assortment of fresh seafood and seaweed caught by the haenyeo in various haenyeo-operated hoetjips (raw fish restaurants) across the island.

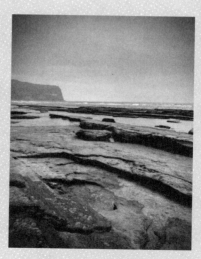

SEE UNTOUCHED LANDSCAPES
OF MOLTEN ROCK

Daily Habits for Longevity

"How old would you be if you didn't know how old
you were? Age is a question of mind over matter.
If you don't mind, it don't matter."

—*Muhammad Ali*

In Bordentown, New Jersey, a Korean farmer named Steve Kwang owns and operates a family farm named after his daughter, Lani. I discovered Lani's Farm at my local GrowNYC greenmarket, where Mr. Kwang's unusually handsome ginger roots first caught my eye. They were markedly different from the dried-up versions languishing at the supermarket, positively bursting with juice, with skin that glowed in pink-yellow hues and thick, bright green stems. I was amused to be so taken with mere ginger roots I began to use them often, whole with the peel on, in my teas and as a base for my soups and other meals at home. I began researching the qualities of ginger root and would later discover that this fresh, young ginger contained about twice as many polyphenols and two to three times more antioxidation activity than the mature ginger found in most grocery stores. After weeks of going back to purchase Mr. Kwang's ginger, I became curious to know more about its origins. So, after an email exchange with the farmer, I drove an hour from the city to visit him.

At sixty, Mr. Kwang was a sprightly figure, his tanned skin and kind eyes shaded under a baseball cap. He explained to me that he had immigrated to the US with his father and sister and that they had started this family farm together when he was seventeen. Every morning, after religiously sleeping a good eight hours and having breakfast (his favorite was doenjang jjigae), he sets out for a full day together with his sister, Eugena, who is sixty-two, to actively run their enterprise. Mr. Kwang is known as the vegetable whisperer. Chefs from all over New York come to him to purchase his distinctively beautiful produce. His sister travels to and from Korea to buy machinery, kitchenware, and sea salt straight from the motherland while running a side business of tiny carnivorous plants, which she sells at the markets in fascinating pots. In their sixties, Mr. Kwang and his sister focus on ambitiously scaling their operations with no signs of retirement. Every day, the two work together to come up with innovative solutions—from reinvesting in the soil to cultivate healthy microbes by taking in kitchen compost, manure, and leftover wood chips from nearby businesses, to finding a bevy of greenhouse solutions to overcome shortages in the harsh winters and beginning their own large inventory of fermented goods and health products like bitter melon powder for diabetics. In a nod to the environmentally friendly ways of the past, they are adamant about keeping the farm eco-conscious and chemical-free. Their lives are filled with the passion of their entrepreneurial spirit and a commitment to growing and selling products of the highest quality, and it shows in the radiance and robustness of the plants they bring to life.

When it was lunchtime, Mr. Kwang invited me to dine at home with his wife and two friends. We sat for a homemade Korean meal with the many components I would come to know as the traditional "longevity" meals of Korea. This one was made of mandu guk (Korean dumpling soup), three types of kimchi, and a potato dish made of kabocha, goguma (Korean sweet potato), and pumpkin, all tossed with spicy gochujang. Mandu guk, when made with tteok (Korean rice cakes), is typically reserved for special occasions like the New Year to wish the recipient good fortune, luck, and prosperity. It was a special day, as the farmer's friends had brought their homemade kimchi to share with their friends. I was so touched that they had invited me in, even though we had just met, to share their food like family. As the Buddhist nuns had taught me, I took each bite thinking about how much time and effort went into aging the kimchi and growing the produce tucked into the mandu—that this is how love is passed on in my culture from one generation to the next and was now a part of me.

After lunch, Mr. Kwang gave me a full tour of the farm, and his sister plucked a plump fig from the tree to feed me again. Sure enough, when we came upon one of the open fields, there was the ssukgat that I craved all the time now. It grew tall, glistening in the sun, its leaves robust and emitting a sweet fragrance that filled the air between us.

Healthy lifespans in Asia

After two decades of living in Asia, I have witnessed firsthand how the elderly in Asian cultures seem to disprove notions of what is achievable at an older age. Many of the elderly that I regularly encounter stridently defy their old age and show traits of those far younger, including astonishingly smooth skin without wrinkles, flexible joints, thick hair, good vision, physical strength, and lower rates of chronic illness. Before my hospital episode, it never occurred to me to look into why this was so.

Since the United Nations began issuing a yearly ranking of projected life expectancy by country, Asian countries have jostled for the number one spot. For decades, Japan led the ranks, sitting staunchly on top of the world's longevity index; their highest concentration of centenarians lives in the sleepy village of Ogimi in Okinawa. Then, in 2015, the densely packed metropolis of Hong Kong overtook Japan and has been holding first place ever since. Researchers now project that South Korea will soon take its turn topping the world charts by 2030, with Korean women expected to live to over ninety years old and Korean men over eighty-four.

The elderly in Korea, Japan, and Hong Kong may differ in the local foods they eat, but they share many of their secrets to maintaining a healthy lifespan and a culture of community that supports a food as medicine lifestyle, which includes daily activity, in particular outdoors. Whether in rural areas or cities like Seoul or Hong Kong, their day-to-day and working lives incorporate nearby mountainsides and beaches, where they can swim in the open waters and hike freely, even during lunch breaks.

As I walked the streets of Seoul, where the largest population of Korea's centenarians live,[1] and observed that many of the elderly were out and about in hiking gear or energetically walking together through the long train tunnels and city streets, I found myself deeply missing my grandparents.

When I was a child, on summer holiday trips from Brooklyn to Korea, my grandparents, who lived in Busan, would take me and my siblings on long walks high into the mountains and then back down to the small villages below. As children, we would get so tired that my grandparents would end up piggybacking us while chatting away, their arms still strong and their minds sharp even with age. Busan was known for its seafood. On these visits, we would play in its coastal seasides and eat fish so fresh they were practically still squirming on the table. For my grandparents, there was always something to be joyful about or something new to learn. As I look back on those memories, I am reminded of how I want to live as I age—looking toward inspiring role models who remained active throughout their lives, sustaining the ways in which so many generations before me thrived.

Redefining old age

Having realized that Korea, Japan, and China shared many wellness philosophies, I kept traveling back and forth between these countries. If I could find overlapping patterns, they might allow me to outline the healthy habits that would support a vibrant, long life. This time, I decided to travel to Ogimi, located on the Japanese island of Okinawa, and estimated at the time to maintain the densest population of centenarians. There, I came upon a stone facing the sea engraved with gold letters: "At 80 years old, I am still a child. When heaven calls for you at 90, say, 'Go away and come back when I am 100.'" This declaration, as fearless and carefree as Peter Pan, was the prevailing pattern that I came to see time and time again on my journey—that what many consider, as I once did, to be the start of decline is really a period of vibrant living in Asia.

When I visited the village of Ogimi, I met a woman in her seventies—a baby, considering the village's longevity declaration. She was toned like an athlete, stunningly wrinkle-free, and dressed casually like a teenager, wearing a T-shirt and jeans with a bandanna on her head. She moved with ease, like a gazelle waiting to spring, and I marveled at her agility. She lived and worked in balmy Ogimi, with its happy-go-lucky ambiance of slower-paced island life. She, like the other residents in Ogimi, consistently kept to their schedules, being active outdoors during the day, which helped their metabolism and circadian rhythms. They enjoyed the pure and traditional foods of their childhood, resting on the same preventative lifestyle and food as medicine philosophy as Korea's yak sik dong won. I would meet many more like her in Asia—individuals of an older age with extraordinary health and moving through life with grace. They eventually upended my views on what aging could mean in my own life.

The greatest common denominator among the youthful seniors I observed was that they spent most of their time outside their homes—even into their one hundreds. When they are not sleeping, they are moving and active all day. In rural areas, they sell what they make and grow, they care for their neighbors, and for most of the day, they engage in physical labor, from farming to fishing to gardening, activities akin to lifting weights and otherwise staying fit and strong. And though they do not typically exercise for exercise's sake, their active lifestyles allow them to maintain flexibility, mobility, and joint strength, whether kneeling to sit on floor mats for meals or squatting while tending their gardens. In the cities, they use public parks to meet, gain a reprieve from the stresses of modern city life, and exercise, many displaying incredibly eye-opening flexibility and strength despite their older age. I saw them all work purposefully and actively engage in social and family activities—a critical line of support as they age.

This image of many of the elderly in Asia—socializing, exercising, and spending time out in nature—is quite different from the idea of senior citizens sitting idly. I realized that these individuals hadn't discovered some magical fountain of youth: Their secret lies in simply embracing a different mentality about older age that gives truth to the adage: "You are only as old as you think you are." In these long-life

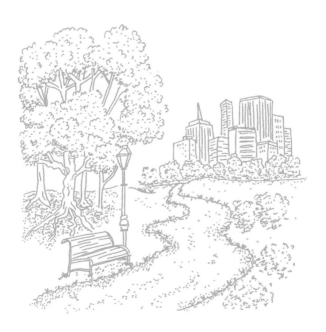

cultures, everyone embraces the outlook that it is important to keep both body and mind active for as long as possible, no matter how old you are. According to "Mama" Cheng Li, my friend's centenarian grandmother, who you'll read about later, staying actively engaged with family and playing brain games are her easy tips for a long and happy life.

Our family had our own near centenarian, who was known for his intelligence and originality. Every morning, he went out, even in the dead of winter, to do cold-water ocean swimming, then back inside for a simple breakfast of walnuts, seaweed, Chinese-style steamed fish, rice, and lightly cooked vegetables which he ate every day. When I first heard about his daily wellness routine, it seemed eccentric to me, but I realized later that he was creating his own approach to stay healthy and strong for as long as he could. He had adopted a healthy way of living that was his own—part wisdom that was passed down, part his own thinking.

Observing the elderly of Asia was truly inspiring and provided a model for the way I hope to live as I get older—enjoying life to its fullest with strength, purpose, and lucidity and dancing through my sunset moments. Of course, it's not really about how long you live, but rather the quality of it. They are proof that it is entirely possible to continue living with purpose into our seventies, eighties, nineties, and one hundreds, rather than reaching older age with expectations, and perhaps feelings of helplessness, of disability. I started to look at the arc of my lifespan with renewed optimism, full of ideas of what I could and wanted to achieve now that I understood that I could have much more time to do them. It was like someone had lifted a veil from my eyes, and I was seeing the full possibilities of my life for the first time.

Wellness cemented by community

When I first moved from the US to Hong Kong, I found it curious to see elderly groups gathering to do extremely slow exercises in the early hours of the morning. I later found out that they were doing tai chi, a traditional Chinese form of martial arts that works on core strength through dynamic movements. On one of my walks, I was also shocked to see a sweet grandmother fiercely wielding a sword for exercise with a friend. And on long-haul flights on Korean airlines, I often saw groups of older passengers watching stretching videos together and devotedly engaging in the recommended exercises to avoid circulation problems caused by extended sitting. As time passed, I would see many other seniors gathering to exercise in a similar fashion. I realized it was the act of remaining active—together—that gave them purpose and cemented these wellness routines to prolong their health spans.

It is well documented that social support and community are key factors for longevity. The value of family and connection is deeply embedded in Asian culture, and seniors in Asia are highly encouraged to maintain active lifestyles, to spend time outdoors, and to maintain vibrant social ties to their community. Support from their family units is provided, growing out of a deep cultural sense of respect and filial responsibility. For example, among many family traditions, Korea observes three separate holidays in May as a reminder of the importance of family: Parents' Day, Grandparents' Day, and Children's Day. In Hong Kong, Qingming Festival, or Tomb Sweeping Day, is meant for families to show respect to their ancestors by sweeping their graves and providing food offerings. In Asia, family and their elderly are considered an important and viable aspect of the social construct of society.

In public parks across Asia, seniors happily congregate for fresh air and a wide variety of activities that engage the body and the brain. I have seen many seniors meet as early as 5:30 a.m. in outdoor spaces near food markets so they can purchase fresh vegetables when the markets open. There are also evening groups that meet after dinner. These group activities give seniors a routine to their days and a reason to wake up happily with meaning and purpose. They require no special equipment or outside expense and therefore are inclusive and accessible to everyone.

There was so much variety to the physical activities I witnessed that at times I couldn't believe my eyes, which had been unaccustomed to the elderly so actively engaged. These activities included:

- Dancing with complex choreography, such as flamenco and ballroom
- Sports encouraging balance and coordination, like badminton, tennis, and basketball
- Physical practices promoting strength and flexibility, like stretching or tai chi, a slow and gentle martial arts form
- Games to stimulate the brain, like card games and mahjong, played with tiles and similar to poker
- Using brightly colored public exercise equipment to climb monkey bars or do planks
- Other physical activities we typically associate with youth, like speed-walking, rollerblading, kite flying, swimming, biking, and playing Hacky Sack and yo-yo
- A very active walking habit, which extends to mountain hikes, barefoot walks, and running errands

Based on what I saw in Asia, it was clear that community, and doing things with others, helped to cement daily habits for wellness. I began to walk more with loved ones, tracking our steps with simple pedometers or Apple Watches. And we began to go out for hikes, spending more

> **Do as the centenarians do**
> - Live with purpose
> - Connect with community
> - Stay active
> - Eat unprocessed local and seasonal foods
> - Drink clean water

time together outside in nature. I walk as much as I can, even intentionally getting out blocks earlier at the train station. And I found that walking within sixty to ninety minutes after dinner almost daily to be a sustainable practice. I also joined group yoga classes both in Hong Kong and New York, positive communities that supported my well-being and encouraged me to go daily. And, finally, I found classes online to restart the creative pursuits of my youth and test my brain, including doodling and playing the piano. These were small first steps but impactful changes that really did help to cement these daily practices for me, and I did end up feeling, as the centenarians do, like a baby, healthier and happier, aging backward.

Successful aging

Deep in many science labs, there is a flurry of research being devoted to unlocking the mysteries of longevity and finding ways to extend our health span, a term that is defined as the period in one's life unburdened by chronic diseases and age-related conditions like arthritis, vision loss, and cognitive decline. Tech billionaires have poured money into finding the magic elixir through advances in biotechnology and drug discovery. Some researchers are focusing on attacking aging in humans through the treatment of old cells. Others are finding how to create lab-grown food to feed our world. Everyone appears to be looking for the holy grail to age well.

Given the billions invested in these efforts, it is fascinating to note that many of the elderly in Asia have achieved long life through natural means, within relatively low-tech environments, and in many cases living in communities removed from modern society. They are not taking pills, or dieting, or avoiding entire food groups. Their holy grail lies in the combination of outdoor exercise, community, and consuming whole, natural foods that are grown on their lands. What this tells us is that the treatments developed in these labs should represent the last mile in healthcare. Longevity begins with preventing disease and maintaining health through lifestyle choices that are as old as time.

Our cells are the workhorses that engine our bodies to function properly. When we intake food and digest it, the cells do the work of taking the nutrients from our food and converting them into energy so that we can function. Our systems are working effectively when the cells continue to divide, making fresh cells to replenish the older ones, which are then eventually removed from our bodies. When this system becomes broken early, premature aging occurs; the cells stop dividing and instead of being removed, they accumulate in our bodies, causing inflammation. When we prevent this from happening, we achieve what scientists call successful aging, which includes freedom from disease and disability, high cognitive and physical functioning, and social and productive engagement, much like what I have seen many centenarians achieving in Asia.

According to the World Health Organization, adherence to a healthy diet and lifestyle can help to prevent many chronic illnesses, such as heart disease. Thus, despite the genetic cards that have been dealt to us, we can all try to achieve successful aging, as these centenarians do, if we just follow the simple mechanics of feeding our bodies the very basic elements required to work effectively. Barring circumstances like physical trauma or a serious health condition, all that is needed for a first step toward prevention are simple low-tech solutions; optimism, healthy food, daily movement, adequate rest cycles, and emotional support of your community are many of the basic "medicines" and ingredients to follow the recipe for a long and healthy life. Sometimes it's the simplest solutions that really are the most elegant and the most effective, and sometimes they can be overlooked and forgotten. Centenarians remind us that we can control how we get older and still be purposeful.

So, if you think your life is coming to a close after a bright youth, consider these key figures in our history, extraordinary individuals who continued their seminal work well past the second half of their century: Thomas Edison, the consummate inventor, who continued inventing breakthroughs well into his eighties; Charlie Chaplin's seventy-five-year acting career; painter Georgia O'Keeffe, who turned to sculpting when she became blind in her eighties and continued her work until ninety-five; Nelson Mandela, who emerged after twenty-seven years in jail to become his country's president at seventy-six; or Julia Child, who was fifty when she hosted her first TV show. And in our family, my own mother surprised us by going back to school in her forties after raising my siblings and me. She managed to win a scholarship to attend the mathematics graduate program at New York University and soon after began teaching high school students, which she continues to do to this day. These individuals, and the centenarians in Asia, inspire me to continue fulfilling my dreams and new ones, too, through my golden years. They remind me that I have so much more to give throughout my life if I take care of my body and my mind.

In Ogimi, while centenarians are thriving, the habits and lifestyle patterns of the younger generation illustrate what happens when the fast pace of modern life begins to usurp the wisdom of traditional life. In Korea, this is known as pali-pali. In Ogimi, younger residents are eager to leave the city's quiet and small economy behind for the promise of better opportunities elsewhere. They move to modern cities like Tokyo, where job opportunities are plentiful and where they often adopt unhealthy and stressful lifestyles, with diets filled with convenient packaged foods. It is becoming common for the older generations remaining in Ogimi to outlive their children who have left, a fact that confirms that longevity is not just related to genetics but deeply tied to diet and lifestyle. While this trend in Ogimi is alarming, it is also a reminder that we can all empower ourselves to live healthfully, no matter our location or budget. It's also a reminder that as we speed into our futures, we should remember to heed the wisdom that our elders have passed down to us. Their tried-and-true methods, which have worked for the generations that came before us, should be considered in tandem with new science. **Modern advances and technology are compatible with traditional practices. The centenarians in Asia are proof of that.**

Korean hygiene for longevity

According to the World Health Organization's definition of self-care, longevity and well-being are also directly related to good hygiene. Roughly a quarter of all human diseases and death in the world can be attributed to environmental factors, including unsafe drinking water, poor sanitation, and personal and general hygiene.[2] Simple measures like handwashing before meals are recommended to stave off illness, and nowhere is good hygiene more apparent than in Korea, where it is taken seriously.

According to a 2019 study involving over 160,000 subjects in South

Korea, improved oral hygiene was associated with a lower risk of irregular heartbeat and heart failure.[3] In Korea, the 3–3–3 brushing method is encouraged; brushing three times per day, within three minutes after having a meal, and for at least three minutes each time. At Samsung, one of the biggest electronic conglomerates in Korea, where I interned as a college student, employees brought their own toothbrush and toothpaste sets, placing them at office desks or lining them up on the sink counters of office bathrooms. It was common to see everyone brush right after lunch.

Another fascinating observation to this American at Samsung was their shoe policy. To help keep office floors clean, all workers would change their outdoor shoes for indoor slippers upon arrival. When I attended internal meetings, I often smiled to myself at the sight of a senior executive who always looked like he'd stepped out of an Adidas commercial, wearing rubber soccer slides with socks. The same holds true at Korean schools. Korean students are taught to treat their schools as their homes, wearing slippers or inside shoes at school. And while employed janitors tend to major cleanup jobs, the students are responsible for cleaning their schools. After school, they use brooms, vacuums, and cloths to clean the classrooms, bathrooms, and other school spaces.

South Koreans care a lot about the cleanliness of their environments too. The streets are spotless, with no visible trash. They also operate well-oiled recycling programs and have tackled waste management effectively with almost zero food waste. Through a mandatory composting scheme, residents squeeze out moisture after filling three-liter food waste bags, priced at 20 cents, to throw away uneaten food, which is then recycled into animal feed or fertilizer. Regimented sorting by both individuals and government, compliance, and frequency of collection have all led to a well-working recycling system that keeps their trash at bay.

Growing up, we always took off our shoes before entering our home, and I never gave much thought to the origins of this practice. But it stems from tradition. Our ancestors needed to keep their floors and their spaces clean, as they slept on the floors with mats and sat on them with low tables to eat. Hygienic practices were a method for keeping illness away, good habits that kept them healthy and living longer.

Longevity Meals

"When you have the best and tastiest ingredients, you can cook very simply and the food will be extraordinary because it tastes like what it is."

—*Alice Waters, chef and public policy advocate for universal access to organic foods*

I wish that I had asked more questions before the matriarchs of my family passed away, that I had soaked up even more of their wisdom when I was with them. These smart women were talented cooks, known for bringing the whole family together for celebrations that featured a delicious array of Korean and Chinese dishes. They also cooked special dishes to nurse family members back to health from colds, surgeries, or postpartum ailments and confinement periods. Growing up as an American, I expected love to be demonstrated through words and hugs. But these women were of a stoic generation, maintaining steely exteriors. Now I understand that for them, they radiated their affections through the way they nourished their loved ones with thoughtfully prepared food.

When I think of them, I try to imagine them at my age and all the things they did so I could try to embody our cultural traditions more fully. I like to think of them nodding in approval if they were with me today, as my memories of them guide me on my journey to rediscover what I had lost of the well-being traditions and my cultural identity. When I think of those family members who are no longer with me, I often reflect on the deeply moving autobiographical essay published by Korean author Chang-rae Lee in the *New Yorker*, "Coming Home Again." Lee achingly recalls the year he spent with his dying mother, resurrecting the Korean dishes of his childhood to feed her during her last days. This is the Asian way—to show your love through food.

Through my travels, I often observed that there was nothing fancy about meals that sustained long-living populations—no artisanal touches or expensive ingredients to define their meals. It was the purity of what was served that struck me most vividly. There was an unabashed simplicity in the presentation of the meals. It wasn't about fancy cooking techniques but rather the high quality of local ingredients, naturally avoiding processed foods.

Simple family meals, cooked thoughtfully to heal and nourish, as my grandmothers and others in my family had done, are what I like to call the longevity meals of Asia. In Korea, longevity meals use principles that date back to the days when the king's physicians and cooks worked together to create healthful royal cuisine (see page 43).

Back in the Joseon Dynasty, the royal cuisine was far more complex, composed of three main tables, plus a separate table for hot pot. The combined tables contained ssukgat; twelve banchan; white rice and red rice with beans; miyeokguk (a rich broth made with seaweed and meat); doenjang (fermented bean paste stew with mixed vegetables and meat); jang (fermented condiments that include light soy sauce, vinegared soy sauce, vinegared red pepper paste, mustard, and salted shrimp juice); grilled skewers; a pan-fried casserole dish; different kinds of kimchi; boiled beef brisket; tricolored cooked vegetables; mung bean jelly salad; braised chicken in soy sauce; pickled pollack roe; dried pollack fluff; dried yellow corvina; raw abalone; poached eggs; and tea.

Today, a typical Korean meal is far simpler but still comprises similar plant-diverse components eaten with golgoru, shared family-style. You could also re-create the principles of this type of longevity meal by creating diversity on your plate or bowl with small portions of various dishes, along with a soup. Often on a busy day, I adopt something I have seen many Korean families do at home—I create a satellite of casually opened banchan-filled jars on the table to share and choose from.

Eating for longevity starts young in Asia

In Korea, children are taught about good nutrition and self-care from the earliest age possible, which contributes to the country's longevity

Elements of a longevity meal

Traditional

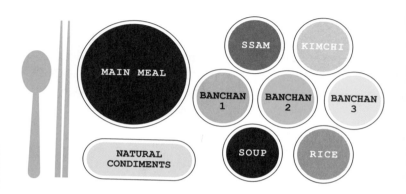

Modified

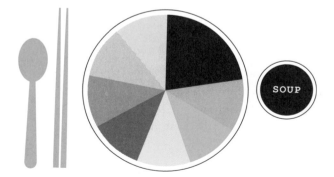

rates. A balanced diet of plant-diverse foods, carbohydrates, and proteins is introduced early on. Highly nutritious foods, like seaweed and kimchi (typically with the spices washed off for young children unaccustomed to the heat), are introduced in small amounts to babies when they are ready to start solids, around six months of age. Korean parents use healthy culinary treatments as a first course of action for minor aches and pains in children, offering broth to keep colds at bay or rice porridge for tummy aches, thereby introducing the concept of food as medicine early. For these little ones, gut health is established very early on, helping to build the bacteria diversity that creates immunity resilience and preventing illness. As they grow up, these early lessons are then supported in school cafeterias, work canteens, and other public places. School lunch trays in Korea will typically include three banchan, along with kimchi, soup, and rice. You will even see this on flights with Korean airlines, where their food trays have multiple divisions to encourage plant-diverse meals.

Chef Jamie Oliver, a passionate advocate who raises awareness about healthy food, calls for increasing "food literacy" in the fight for our health and our planet. Food literacy is about empowering ourselves, and our children, with the knowledge to make healthy food choices. For children, being able to identify a healthy ingredient like a tomato from ketchup, its processed version, and cooking with parents at home, are big parts of the equation of food literacy. According to educational studies, children retain 25 percent of what they listen to, 45 percent of what they listen to and see, and 70 percent when they practice what they are learning hands-on. It also follows that in addition to teaching young children about nutrition, we must also begin teaching them to cook and prepare food from an early age.

In Hong Kong, where I live, the food as medicine philosophy is embraced from an early age too. Their family-style meals feature a diverse array of vegetables, cooked with small pieces of chopped sea-food or meat. Hong Kong residents don't typically have the space to grow their own produce, but within each of its eighteen districts is a dedicated farmer's market, which translates to a walking distance of less than twenty minutes no matter where you live. Hong Kong, with its city lights and fast-paced culture, may seem the polar opposite of what one might find in the rural areas where many centenarians live. However, residents in both rural areas and cities who follow traditional ways are apples that fall from the same tree.

My Hong Kong friend Therese's grandmother is fondly referred to by her family as Mama. Mama is a centenarian who has been profiled in the local newspaper, known for preparing traditional Chinese meals at home, using little oil and fresh ingredients devoid of preservatives, col-orings, additives, sugar, dairy, or fried foods. She eats in moderation with a light breakfast of boiled congee or a slice of toast; lunch and dinner are either steamed fish, homemade tofu, or blanched chicken with vegeta-bles and rice. Other ingredients featured in her meals include pickled vegetables, bone broth, dried scallops, shrimp, mushrooms, orange peel, sweet dates, lotus seeds, peanuts, red dates, white fungus, almonds, bok choy, dried figs, and sea cucumbers. Mama cooks with spontaneity. Her dishes are modern heirlooms, passed down through generations in her family and adjusted with her own tips and tricks.

The best ingredients you can find

At the heart of building a longevity meal is a solid foundation of the best plant-based ingredients that you can find, and as many of them as you can include over a single day. This is one of the secrets from long-living cultures, many of whom grow their food or have fresh ingredients easily accessible to them. It doesn't mean buying the most expensive ingredients—it means buying fresh. If you can, choosing mostly local and seasonal produce is optimal because these ingredients have not degraded in nutrient levels on a plane or truck ride to get to you (while also taking a more sustainable carbon-neutral approach), but also because you are choosing it in its peak ripeness and flavor. Sometimes you can't do this because you want that avocado that isn't grown in your city, or that blueberry you want in your daily diet but isn't in season where you live. The best ingredients can also involve finding things in powdered or dried form, like sun-dried shiitake mushrooms or blue-green algae, as well as in frozen form as I often choose for wild berries when I can't find them fresh. As Michelin-star chef Alice Waters once said: "I dare you to cut open a selection of fresh fruit, and serve it." When you have a high-quality, fresh ingredient like a watermelon bursting with flavor, sometimes all the meal entails is just eating it fresh (as nature intended for you to have it), in all of its natural deliciousness.

I finally started to cook

You may be surprised to learn that before I started on this healing journey, the idea of stepping into the kitchen to prepare a meal felt quite daunting. I relied on takeout, convenience foods, and eating out at restaurants. However, as I took cooking classes and began to re-create the traditional dishes of my heritage, I realized that healthy cooking doesn't need to be elaborate or perfect. I no longer follow instructions to a tee for my favorite recipes. Instead, using the philosophy that I learned from the Buddhist nuns called uhmuni's sohn maht, I simply adjust to taste or improvise by substituting for leftover ingredients to take a zero-waste approach. Even if I find a modern invention that will make cooking easier, like a ready-made broth base or tea packet, I always try to make a healthy recipe from scratch at least once so I understand how it is made. This has also allowed me to understand the purpose of a recipe's ingredient—for example, how a jujube naturally sweetens a soup, or which ingredients aren't all that necessary, like an artificial preservative to promote a food's shelf life.

As I gained confidence, cooking dinner became a family affair in our home. The kids would help me to prepare our simple dinners by washing, cutting, and stirring ingredients. They started to voice their preferences on ingredients, and I could see that they enjoyed going with me to the market to forage for new menu items. We even had family cooking competitions to see who could come up with the best dishes.

Some of the ingredients I discovered, like specific citrus fruits or seaweeds, were not available where I lived, but I was able to find suitable alternatives. Seaweeds, like nori, wakame, and kombu, are now part of my regular routine, and I add small amounts of these to broths and salads, and I snack on dried seaweed sheets.

Lemons too became part of my every day. I squeeze fresh lemon into my water or as a finishing touch to almost any dish. I also peel and freeze the rind, where most of the nutrients are, to add to recipes later. Not only do we enjoy the delicious touch of acidity in our meals, but we are reaping the benefits of additional antioxidants and vitamin C. I start my day before yoga class with a small cup of a drink that emulates the electrolyte-filled Gatorade, but without the refined sugar or artificial sweetener—warm water, a pinch of salt, and a squeeze of half a lemon, sometimes with a slice of fresh ginger with the peel on. When you sleep, you lose water and electrolytes, which I replace by drinking this simple concoction. The combination of drinking the lightly salted water, which is warm and gentle on the stomach, along with the vitamin C in the lemon, has done wonders to bring back the salt, electrolytes, and water, the flush of rosiness in my face, my energy levels, and my performance in yoga class.

I also started incorporating the healthy carbohydrates and proteins I had discovered. I added purple and black rice to meals, and sweet potatoes, which I bake and eat with the peel on. For protein, I now cook more fish and fermented bean soups, doenjang and miso, on a weekly basis. Natto—and other fermented soybeans, which are the bedrock of longevity meals in Korea, Japan, and China—was another way for me to get beans in while having more probiotics in my diet. I eat a small amount of natto dressed with whole-grain dijon mustard and persimmon vinegar or soy sauce along with my breakfast, and sometimes as a topping for salads, rice dishes, and soups. One heaping spoonful of natto, which tastes mild and earthy, provides high levels of bone-healthy vitamin K and probiotics.

Like the Koreans do, I decided to improve the quality of our water and purchased a filtration system that connects to the faucet. It was easy to install, and we now get water free of chlorine, nitrates and nitrites, and heavy metals for home cooking and drinking. I also bought a non-plastic, temperature-controlled, electric water heater, which heats up my water in minutes for tea at home. I have a second one in the office for making tea at work. Purified water is key in many of our family meals, which now include nutritional Korean guk and stews for a main meal or as a side dish.

I am now much more adventurous to try new things that promote wellness, and for fun, I might experiment with a supplement or a new powder. At a visit to a detox spa, I was instructed to have one digestive aid supplement a day, which I have found to be helpful. I tend to take these once a day with dinner and when I travel, but I have come to know that many of these more modern wellness hacks are optional; what isn't optional are real foods, and I also make sure that I take in as many naturally occurring enzymes and nutrients from real foods as possible.

Doenjang jjigae (fermented bean stew)

Jiggaes became a new kind of breakfast for me. They are fairly simple to prepare and staples in Korean kitchens. Doenjang jjigae is made with fermented soybean paste and filled with plants and protein from the tofu. This dish is flavorful and comforting and has become my daughter's favorite Korean dish, as it was in my childhood too. I tend to make meatless versions for her in the mornings, as we do bigger meat dishes when the entire family can all sit together at dinnertime. She loves them served with a little rice and cut roasted seaweed on top.

Recipe notes

For my quick version of doenjang, I add the doenjang paste when the heat is very low so as to keep the probiotics alive and beneficial for the gut in the soup. As I mentioned before, exposing live probiotic cultures to temperatures above 120°F kills them.

Tofu comes in a variety of textures, ranging from very soft to firm. My preference is for the soft version.

INGREDIENTS

Serves 2

1 tablespoon olive oil

1 tablespoon minced garlic

⅓ medium onion, minced

2 cups anchovy broth (see page 116) or filtered water

1 small green or red chili

1 medium zucchini, cut into 1-inch cubes

2 tablespoons doenjang (Korean soybean paste)

1 block soft-textured tofu, cut into 1-inch cubes

1 teaspoon white or fruit-based vinegar (optional)

1 scallion, greens roughly sliced, whites saved for the soup

METHOD

1. In a small pot, heat the oil over medium heat. Add garlic and onion and cook until translucent, 5 to 10 minutes.

2. In a medium pot, combine the anchovy broth and chili and bring to a boil over high heat.

3. Add the zucchini and cook until it is soft, about 5 minutes.

4. Turn the heat down to very low heat, add the doenjang paste, and stir until thoroughly mixed. Add the tofu, then turn off heat.

5. Add the vinegar and scallions, then cover to lightly cook with the residual heat of the soup.

Fermented soybeans: The bedrock of longevity meals in Korea, Japan, and China

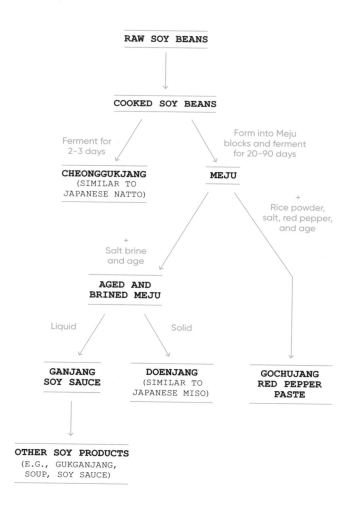

RAW SOY BEANS

↓

COOKED SOY BEANS

Ferment for 2-3 days ↙   ↘ Form into Meju blocks and ferment for 20-90 days

CHEONGGUKJANG
(SIMILAR TO JAPANESE NATTO)

MEJU

+ Rice powder, salt, red pepper, and age

+ Salt brine and age ↙

AGED AND BRINED MEJU

Liquid ↙   Solid ↘

GANJANG SOY SAUCE

DOENJANG
(SIMILAR TO JAPANESE MISO)

GOCHUJANG RED PEPPER PASTE

↓

OTHER SOY PRODUCTS
(E.G., GUKGANJANG, SOUP, SOY SAUCE)

A new order of eating

In a traditional Korean longevity meal, food is served in an order that aids digestion and yields the greatest health benefits. Banchan, sides that include vegetable dishes and fermented foods like kimchi, is always served first, before the main meal. Protein and carbohydrates come after, then fruits and anything sweet later. The optimal time to eat fermented foods is at the beginning of the meal, so that they can do the work of helping digestion as soon as they land in the stomach. The order of the traditional longevity meal is backed by modern science as well. According to a study published in the *Diabetes Care* journal, blood sugar spikes, which can lead to irreversible inflammation like diabetes, can be reduced by 75 percent by eating high-fiber vegetables first, followed by proteins and fats, with carbohydrates coming last, all of which helps to slow down the digestion of simple carbohydrates and sugars.[1] I adopted this way eating, beginning each meal with fermented foods and vegetable dishes. I make this easy by keeping sauerkraut, kimchi, or a prepared vegetable dish, like roasted brussels sprouts, in my fridge at all times, to eat a bit first before tucking in to my meals.

Our stomachs are most sensitive to absorbing and processing carbohydrates and sugars, even in fruits, when they are empty. Eating a sugar- or carb-heavy meal on an empty stomach will immediately result in blood sugar level spikes and crashes, which we want to avoid. This is why I switched from eating sugary cereals and pastries for breakfast to traditional Korean or otherwise Asian-style breakfasts. Now, I like to start my day with one or two tablespoons of a fermented dish with a splash of vinegar, followed by a savory plant-based breakfast with protein that might include a Korean guk, dinner leftovers from the refrigerator, miso soup with seaweed and tofu, cottage cheese with produce, rice with salmon, curry, or a quick omega-3-rich canned skipjack tuna (that is lower in mercury than larger tuna like albacore) with chopped celery and spices. For a beverage, I'll have green tea, matcha, or coffee with no sugar. This is not to say that I don't ever have something like a croissant in the morning, but it's not my mainstay, and I make sure that I have the vinegar-fermented bite beforehand.

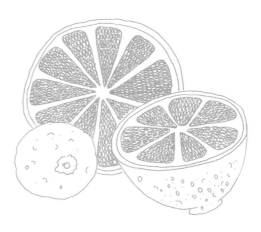

Rediscovering the diversity of our planet

Beyond embracing the whole plant philosophy, we would do well to learn more about the underutilized plant-based food categories that have enormous benefits for human health and for the sustainability of our planet: mushrooms, wild plants, and seaweed. These food groups have been used for centuries in Asia for medicinal and nutritional purposes, but they have yet to fully enter mainstream diets elsewhere.

Take, for example, mushrooms. Although they have incredible health benefits, it is estimated that only 10 percent of mushrooms on the planet have even been identified. Cultivated for centuries for their texture and rich umami flavor, they make a tasty addition to many dishes. They are rich in vitamins B and D, as well as protein and fiber, and they have been linked to reducing allergies, cholesterol, and cancer risk. They can also boost immunity, balance the gut, improve mood and focus, and delay cellular aging.

In traditional Asian cuisine and health remedies, there are many mushroom varieties that are used fresh for cooking as well as in dried form, mainly for teas or tinctures. My favorite fresh mushrooms for cooking are shiitake, snow fungus, cloud ear, and enoki. They are delicious when lightly cooked on their own as a side dish or added to omelets, hot pots, and stir-fries. I use truffle-scented olive oil for special occasions as a deeply fragrant final splash to cooked greens or soup. In Hong Kong, you can buy snow fungus in the markets fresh off the tree trunk; it is known for its skin beautifying properties. When compared to the same amount of broccoli, snow fungus has fifteen times more fiber, a skyrocketing amount of vitamin D, four times more potassium, six times more calcium, more magnesium, and four times more iron. When I am in Hong Kong, I like to make a warm tea with snow fungus steeped with one ginger slice with the skin on, a star anise, and dendrobium orchid root.

Beyond mushrooms, numerous plants that are considered weeds also have great health benefits. Purslane, for example, is actually a potent anti-inflammatory, wound-healing herb with nutritive properties that extends cell life to produce youthful, healthy skin and contains the highest content of vitamin A among green leafy vegetables. Studies have also shown that many of these wild plants have more nutrients than their cultivated versions, like the wild blueberry, which contains more bio-active compounds compared to the cultivated blueberry. Though they are smaller in size, wild blueberries are higher in antioxidants, such as anthocyanins and flavonoids, which are anti-inflammatory.

Wild plants like ssukgat and goji berries play an integral part in many dishes in Asia. These plants have many culinary uses, as they have powerful antioxidant and anti-inflammatory properties, and are delicious. Ssukgat flowers and goji berries can be dried for teas, and their greens can be used for hot pots or lightly blanched as a side. Wild plants often appear ground up in the form of spices, or as dried herbs when we encounter them in grocery stores in modern life. Herbs and spices should be longevity pantry staples.

While there are numerous spices that I use in my cooking, I like to include turmeric, cinnamon, and white pepper every day in my beverages like coffee, and I also use dried basil, rosemary, oregano, and thyme as a finishing touch to Western-style soups. Long used in Asian cuisine, turmeric has powerful anti-inflammatory properties and has been linked to help control diabetes, cholesterol, and arthritis, inhibit cancer cell growth, improve digestion and the immune system, and improve the tautness and radiance of the skin. Turmeric is activated when combined with pepper, which itself helps digestion; its active ingredient, curcumin, has been used traditionally to treat skin disorders, upper respiratory tract disorders, joint pain, digestive problems, and more. Cinnamon acts to lower blood sugar and is also rich in anti-inflammatory properties.

When it comes to herbs, cilantro and parsley are favorites. I like to use them for their detoxification powers and their mild flavors and sprinkle them on as a final layer to many dishes. I use the mint family of herbs like perilla leaves, shiso, and mint as I would a vegetable. And I make small premixed batches of spices and herbs so I can readily use them in the kitchen.

My premade mixes for plant diversity

These three premade mixes are on my version of a lazy Susan because I use them daily.

Recipe notes

Spices do not expire in a way that would make you sick to consume them, but they lose their flavor potency as they pass their peak freshness. Ground spices lose their freshness past six months, while whole spices can last for up to five years.

Korean-inspired salt mix

INGREDIENTS

Equal parts:

yeast extract

kombu seaweed, finely ground with mortar and pestle or spice grinder

miyeok (brown algae or wakame), finely ground with mortar and pestle or a spice grinder

pink Himalayan salt

METHOD

- Combine all the ingredients in a container with a lid and shake to combine.

Yeast extract is rich in amino acids, the building blocks of protein, and I like to use it to flavor dishes like eggs. Sprinkle a small amount on any dish—meat, fish, noodles, or soups—to add a savory zest.

Turmeric–cinnamon pepper mix

INGREDIENTS

Equal parts:
ground turmeric
ground cinnamon
ground white pepper

METHOD

- Combine all the ingredients in a container with a lid and shake to combine.

I like to use white rather than black pepper for its more subtle, mild flavor, especially because I sprinkle this spice mix in my teas and coffee daily.

Seed mix

INGREDIENTS

Equal parts:
black sesame seeds
white sesame seeds
pumpkin seeds
sunflower seeds
chia seeds
flax seeds

METHOD

- Combine all the ingredients in a container with a lid and shake to combine.

I picked up black sesame seeds in my Asian cooking classes. They are rich in omega-3 fatty acids and fiber, like flax seeds.

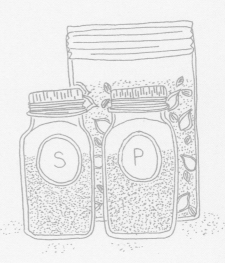

My grandmother's myeolchi (anchovy) broth

Rather than merely serving to flavor the other ingredients in a soup dish, Koreans consider the guk, or broth, as a key ingredient, and will drink the guk even in a ramen noodle soup. In Korean culture, it is incredibly important to include a nutritious and nourishing broth as part of a meal; guk is never a throwaway item.

This broth is the foundation to my favorite meal that my late grandmother used to cook, her doenjang jjigae (see page 109). Her secret was to grind the dried ingredients—the anchovy, the shrimp, and the shiitake mushrooms—by mortar and pestle. Then she would divide them into small pouches and freeze them, using them for her broth as needed.

I like to make this broth on its own to drink out of a mug, and I serve it to the kids when they have colds to speed up their recovery. I have adapted her recipe to include kombu, which adds more nutrition, and I keep store-bought packets of the soup base for when I run out of time or my homemade versions.

Recipe notes

Kombu is mineral-rich, meaning it is high in iodine, essential for thyroid functioning, iron, and calcium, as well as in vitamins A and C. It is a natural flavor and health enhancer that I try to use as a base for all of my soups if I can.

You can make the broth packets ahead of time, as my grandmother did, and freeze them for up to 6 months.

INGREDIENTS

Makes 8 cups

2 large dried shiitake mushrooms

6 dried shrimp (optional)

10 to 12 medium dried anchovies

One 2 x 2-inch piece kombu

Special tool: Soup base pouches, if making your own

METHOD

1. Grind the dried mushrooms, shrimp, if using, and anchovies using a mortar and pestle and stuff them in a cheesecloth packet. Alternatively, you can use a store-bought packet.

2. In a medium pot, combine 8 cups water, the broth packet, and kombu. Bring to a boil over high heat, then cover, reduce the heat, and simmer for 20 minutes.

3. Remove the broth packet and kombu before serving.

Hoedeopbap (raw fish bibimbap, or mixed rice)

This is my son's favorite dish to eat after playing competitive sports. It's filled with healthy protein, carbohydrates, and fat, and loads of nutrients from the variety of fresh produce and other ingredients. The Korean sauce with its mildly spicy gochujang makes this dish really flavorful and delicious. Gochujang is also considered a diet-friendly superfood because it's rich in protein, antioxidants, and vitamins but low in fat and calorie content. And it's the most-requested, easy-to-make recipe in my longevity toolbox that always inspires the question: "Can you please share this recipe with me?"

Recipe notes

Black and red rice contain antioxidants known as anthocyanins—also found in blueberries, grapes, and acai—that have been linked to a decreased risk of heart disease and cancer, improvements in memory, and other health benefits.

Salmon roe and flying fish roe are high in healthy omega-3 fats, which reduce inflammation and support brain and heart health.

INGREDIENTS

Serves 4

1 tablespoon gochujang (red pepper paste)

1 tablespoon rice vinegar

1 tablespoon toasted sesame oil

1 tablespoon mirin

1 tablespoon soy sauce

1 cup cooked rice (I like to mix black, purple, red, and brown rice), warm

½ pound fresh sashimi-grade salmon (feel free to include other fish like tuna or yellowtail), diced

4 to 5 cups mixed greens (soft red lettuces and crunchy romaine), diced

4 perilla leaves, chopped

½ to 1 cucumber, cut into thin matchsticks

¼ carrot, cut into thin matchsticks

1 teaspoon flying fish roe and/or salmon roe

1 packet roasted seaweed snack, cut into thin strips

Sesame seeds, for garnish

METHOD

1. In a large bowl, gently mix the gochujang, vinegar, sesame oil, mirin, and soy sauce, then mix in the more solid ingredients—rice, diced sashimi, mixed greens and perilla leaves—until they are well combined.

2. Arrange the cucumber and carrot on top. Sprinkle with the fish roe, then the seaweed and sesame seeds. Serve immediately.

The Asian heritage food pyramid

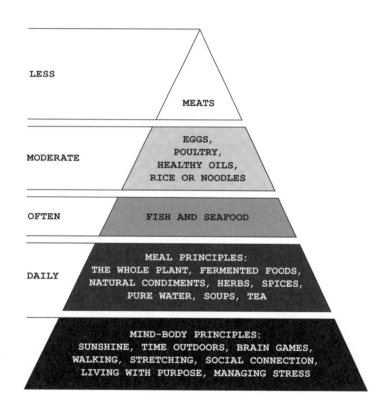

LESS — MEATS

MODERATE — EGGS, POULTRY, HEALTHY OILS, RICE OR NOODLES

OFTEN — FISH AND SEAFOOD

DAILY — MEAL PRINCIPLES: THE WHOLE PLANT, FERMENTED FOODS, NATURAL CONDIMENTS, HERBS, SPICES, PURE WATER, SOUPS, TEA

MIND-BODY PRINCIPLES: SUNSHINE, TIME OUTDOORS, BRAIN GAMES, WALKING, STRETCHING, SOCIAL CONNECTION, LIVING WITH PURPOSE, MANAGING STRESS

The Asian heritage food pyramid

As I started to cook and eat in this new way, I gave more thought to the ingredients that had once been the foundations of my diet, and how this balance had shifted through my travels. I learned that a food and nutrition nonprofit named Oldways had developed the Asian Diet Pyramid in conjunction with the China-Cornell-Oxford Project on Nutrition, Health and Environment and the Harvard School of Public Health. Like the Mediterranean Diet Pyramid, this pyramid for Asia was developed to illustrate traditional diets as models for healthy eating because of the historical low incidence of chronic disease in specific regions across the world. I found the record of these traditional eating habits an inspiring source of information to form a new way to live. I also adapted the Oldways version to mimic more closely what I had found firsthand in Asia, including, for example, concepts for the whole plant and natural condiments.

But food is only one extension of other aspects of a healthy lifestyle. Even today, the official Korean food pyramid includes a base layer for daily mind-body activity and community. For those who subscribe to a food as medicine philosophy, the food we eat is only part of the equation. Equally important is achieving balance in the way that we prepare and consume our food, and in the way that it fuels our bodies. Balance comes in many forms from an Eastern philosophy perspective.

As part of my Asian nutrition training, I took a cooking class at the Black Sesame Kitchen school in Beijing and was surprised to learn from our instructor Sophie that stress management and balance are essential to healthy longevity eating. In Eastern philosophy, balance comes into play in many forms. **At mealtime, according to Eastern philosophy, balance involves building a colorful, seasonal plate that incorporates the five commonly known tastes: bitter, sweet, sour, salty,**

and savory. (Ayurveda includes two more: pungent and astringent.) Foods are also consumed for their nutritional and medicinal value as a course correction for imbalances in the body.

According to Sophie, balance also comes through the physical activities we engage in throughout the day: sleep, rest, stress management, and daily movement. Our body's endocrine system—a network of glands that produce hormones regulating metabolism, growth, and development—is activated by daily movement. This includes building strength and mobility by rising in a controlled movement from the floor after sitting down as the centenarians do, and it is deactivated by a sedentary lifestyle.

In the traditional Asian diet, balance also comes into play in terms of the types of foods that you eat. Asians have long eaten gluten-heavy noodles and high-glycemic white rice without health consequences. The key is in balance and moderation. It isn't about the noodles or the rice; they are mere supplements and small portions that accompany nutrient-dense, high-fiber, and mostly plant-based meals. Studies have shown that the impact of high-glycemic and "inflammatory" foods can be softened by combining them with their opposites, low-glycemic and non-inflammatory foods—for example, a small portion of white rice with kimchi and other vegetables.

The Life-Changing Benefits of Walking

"If you take 100 steps after each meal, you'll live to 99."

—*ancient Chinese proverb*

Soon after I returned from another trip to Korea back to Hong Kong, COVID-19 hit. For many months, we were stuck inside with gyms closed and many people working from home. In an effort to stay healthy while social distancing, I decided to try something simple but novel for me. Like the centenarians, I would venture outside each day to walk.

After meals, I got in the habit of walking down to the beaches near our family's home, listening to the calming crash of waves along the shore. I would walk in the morning to catch the first rays of light, at sunset, and during the evenings when I could watch the night sky filled with luminescent stars with a childlike wonder. When I had more time, I climbed stone staircases to reach hidden trails and forests filled with old banyan trees, with their spindly roots and the sweet aroma of moss and tropical flowers wafting through the air. Every so often, I'd hear a chorus of croaking frogs; a bat would soar above me; or an owl, boar, or possum would appear. These wild things reminded me of the majesty of this world we live in. I would stop to notice everything, even to watch the ladybugs below and the butterflies above. Everything that seemed to matter in the human world lost its importance in the simplicity and beauty of the outdoors. On these walks outside, I felt mindful and alive, in touch with the natural world in a way that I never had before.

In Hong Kong, as in Seoul or Ogimi, walking in the outdoors is common. In a study published in *Nature*, researchers at Stanford examined data from smartphones for ninety-five days and found that Hong Kong residents walk the most of anyone in the world, with a daily average of almost seven thousand steps per day,[1] which is equivalent to a little more than one hour a day. Ever since, Hong Kong's longevity rates have been tied to their steady walking habits. Studies now show that our risk of premature death is reduced the more we walk; human mortality is cut by at least 50 percent by increasing the number of steps we take per day to six thousand to eight thousand for adults aged sixty years and older, and to eight thousand to ten thousand steps per day among adults younger than sixty years.

Walking after meals is an especially effective wellness tool, as walking helps to flatten glucose spikes (a physiological event that happens when glucose builds up in the bloodstream after eating, which if not controlled can lead to weight gain, diabetes, and heart disease). According to a 2022 study published in the journal *Sports Medicine*, light walking for as little as two to five minutes after a meal reduced blood glucose levels by 17 percent compared to prolonged sitting.[2] The American Diabetes Association recommends walking for slightly longer—ten minutes after dinner—to control glucose levels.

Walking also benefits the brain. A 2022 study published in the *Journal of Alzheimer's Disease Reports* revealed that twelve weeks of walking for thirty minutes, four times a week, resulted in improved neural connectivity and memory function in both cognitively healthy older adults and those with cognitive decline.[3] Developing a daily walking practice has significantly changed my metabolism and ability to maintain an optimal weight as no other exercise has before.

Being outdoors also helps to support our body's natural functions. Evolutionarily speaking, we are programmed to be outdoors while the sun is shining, and home in bed when it gets dark at night. Studies demonstrate that we should be outside at least two hours per day to offset myopia, the inability to clearly see far-sighted objects, by being able to see into the distance and being exposed to outdoor light.[4] Walking while being exposed to sunlight and the outdoors, and even the mere sight and sound of water on a sunny day, can help to increase the brain's release of the hormone serotonin, which is associated with boosting mood and helping us feel calm and focused. At night, darker lighting triggers the brain to make another hormone, melatonin, which will help you to sleep.

Walking outdoors is one of the best forms of exercise. It is free, requiring no equipment, and it enables you to reconnect with the natural world, even if it is just by walking in your city while noticing the seasonal changes in trees or hearing the sound of water. Walking thirty minutes to one hour after dinner in the evenings, combined with shorter stints of walking throughout the day, helps to keep me energized and at the fitness performance level that is most optimal for me. It also efficiently fits into my schedule.

When I was in Seoul, I was impressed that the city was so walkable. Walking is enabled through the smart city capabilities like its remarkable public transport. High-tech and easy to use, with trains entirely enclosed within glass doors to keep their tracks clean and to avoid passenger accidents, public transport and technology in Seoul seemed to be directly related to the number of centenarians in the city and their ability to stay healthy and active. Equally impressive, Wi-Fi is available practically everywhere in Seoul, including in trains, and elderly citizens are proficient in using technology and smart public transportation to

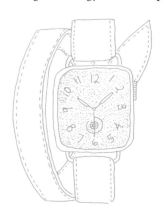

plan their travel and walking routes. As I walked along Seoul's gingko trees on the streets, I realized they were the same gloriously yellow-leafed ones that grow in places like Manhattan's Central Park and Hong Kong. Gingko trees are often planted in cities for their resilience to pollution, a sign of modern times, but they also grow valuable medicine within, used in teas to help blood circulation and memory issues. Gingko trees symbolize long life and prosperity, bidding well wishes for the people passing by. They can live strong for hundreds, even a thousand years, and each fall they shed their uniquely fanned leaves, which twirl down to a golden sea on the ground.

Everyday ways to walk more

- Use a simple pedometer or an Apple Watch
- Set a daily move goal. My daily goal started small, and I gradually increased it as I made progress
- Think about errands and household tasks like vacuuming as contributing to your move goal. Even the most mundane of tasks, like walking to the grocery store, increases your step count, which, for me, provides a dopamine hit and rewards me for achieving this small goal
- If you live in an urban setting, challenge yourself to get off the train before your usual stop, or get off the elevator before your usual floor, and walk the rest of the way
- Pair your walks with something you like, like listening to a podcast or a playlist, or scheduling a phone call with a friend
- Walk with a family member, friend, or other loved one

WATER

Ssukgat flourishes in restorative, hydrating environments. Water of poor quality can be responsible for slow growth, discoloration, and, in some cases, a shorter lifespan. Water that is clean strengthens its growth. Water gives life.

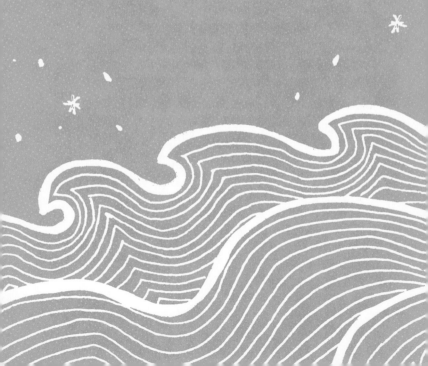

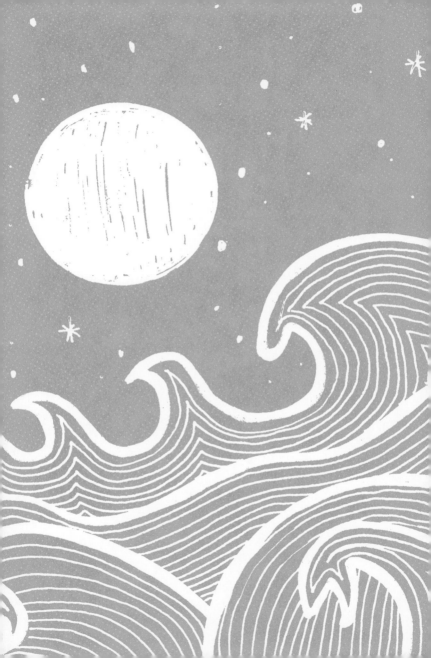

Haenyeo: Stewards of the Sea

"Ieodo sana, ieodo sana, ieodo sana. Where to go,
where to row. All aboard to the depths of the sea.
Where my mother gave birth to me. Did she know to
dive would be my destiny?"

—*Song of the haenyeo*

Fifty miles south of the Korean peninsula, there is a windy little island called Jeju with a dormant volcano looming at its center. Fire-born Jeju formed two million years ago by volcanic eruptions that created an almost otherworldly landscape of molten rock. It is home to residents who yearn for its crystal-clear waters and wild, unbridled nature, much of which remains largely untouched by human hands. For hundreds of years on Jeju, female divers known as haenyeo have darted in and out of the waters along this coastline, catching seafood for their livelihood.

These sea mermaids free dive without oxygen tanks, descending to depths of more than sixty feet while carrying only simple tools: their signature orange floats and green nets, small harpoons for piercing fish, sickles for collecting seaweed, and long hoes for prying abalone from rocks. When they return to land, their nets are filled with sea delicacies fit for fine dining: abalones, conches, sea urchins, octopus, and rare seaweed like hijiki. Haenyeo dive for up to seven hours a day, holding their breath as they dive, resurfacing each time with a unique whistle exhalation known as sumbisori. If you visit Jeju and happen to hear the sound of whistling over the open waves, as I had, that's the haenyeo calling to check on each other, like playful dolphins signaling in the ocean.

Harvesting seafood in this way is extremely challenging, even for the physically strong. Diving at such great depths, repeatedly and for extended lengths of time in cold water, can lead to decompression injuries, heart attack, and death. The haenyeo also contend with dangers such as jellyfish, harsh weather, and sharks. But these women defy any preconceived notions of what is physically achievable, and more so because the average age of haenyeo is over sixty, with the oldest in their eighties. Only the older divers of Jeju have been at it long enough to build up the stamina required to do this job. The haenyeo begin to train at age eleven, going into greater ocean depths as they age and even diving through pregnancies. The oldest haenyeo are the matriarchs of the island, staunch carriers of a tradition that began when there was a need for women to provide income for their families while many of the island's men were lost to deep-sea fishing accidents or wars during the seventeenth century when the gender shift began. The women's higher fat reserves were also thought to make them more resistant to cold water.

When I was growing up, these haenyeo existed for me in stories and books, like folklore. With hard-lined faces, tanned and salted from life at sea, they were always depicted as warriors, revered for their resilience and the nobility of their work. When I went to Jeju to see them for myself, they could not have been more different from the soft, girlish images of K-pop culture. The haenyeo I encountered projected a stoic majesty. They have become symbols of resilience through Korea's hardships and the inadvertent protectors of its ocean environment.

A quick look at the haenyeo and one might consider them brusque or hurried. That was certainly my first impression when I tried to approach them. When they are diving, there is no time for frivolity—their lives are at stake. The haenyeo live within a private subculture, a tightly knit community bonded through their uniquely shared challenges and experiences of life on water. Many of the haenyeo did not choose this way of life; they were born into it. But they have each other and their special sisterhood to fall back on. The haenyeo community ritually gathers around bonfires to form group decisions, share skills, tell stories, and exchange clothes while warming themselves. They work together to collect, dry, and sell their sea gatherings. They take care of one another's babies while the others work. When they retire from diving, they work together at hoetjips, or raw fish restaurants, where they serve dishes made from the day's haenyeo catch, like abalone porridge and vinegared sea cucumbers.

As I turned my back to leave them to their work at the shoreline, I heard their laughter before they burst into song, the simplicity and pure joy of its sound touching my soul deeply.

Guardians of the water

Jeju Island is historically known for its pristine waters, but, increasingly, the haenyeo must dive to extract garbage from the sea, including plastics, fishing nets, and litter. Today, 4,300 haenyeo remain, down from 15,000 when they were a thriving population. Many experts believe this generation of haenyeo will be the last, as the young leave for cities and pollution destroys their place of work. To nurture the sea's ecosystem, they have also become sustainable harvesters, seeding growth for snails and abalone and managing seaweeds to clear rock substrate for the shellfish. They have strict regulations about where, when, and at what size they gather abalone and other marine life to ensure the sustainability of their stock in the ocean, avoiding spawning periods and overharvesting. The haenyeo truly live up to the name bestowed on them, which means "women of the sea," the mothers who guard the vitality of this underworld.

While visiting Jeju, I had the opportunity to try the haenyeo's fresh catch thanks to the Hwang family, who own a regenerative farm, a wellness practice, and a private farm-to-table restaurant on the island. They work with the haenyeo to guard the waters and a way of living that is in sync with nature and the environment. Their restaurant uses only natural, chemical-free ingredients to create specialty items like their in-house fermented condiments—the jangs, twelve-year flavored kimchi, homemade wines, teas, and tofu. Mrs. Hwang, the head chef, and her daughter, Chef Jiwon, help to run the kitchen while daughter Nabee (whose name aptly means "butterfly" in Korean) is trained in traditional Chinese medicine. Mr. Hwang and Nabee travel regularly between Jeju, Seoul, and the US to do research that informs their menu, which is predicated on yak sik dong won, Korea's food as medicine approach. Mr. Hwang chose Jeju Island as a home base for the family's operation precisely because of the healing properties of its clean, mineral-rich water. When Mr. Hwang told me this, I remembered that my father always referred to Jeju as a dreamland where nature abounds.

The Hwangs opened their wellness practice and restaurant after Mr. Hwang was diagnosed with type-2 diabetes and lost his ability to see in one of his eyes. His health crisis led him to become an expert in food and nutritional therapy, utilizing functional food concepts and the medicinal qualities of different foods, and with his wife learning to cook and feed him these foods. Mr. Hwang's story became so well-known that others in Korea sought his advice for personalized diet consultations. He has become known as a self-healing master of sorts and has even mentored chefs like Hooni Kim, the first Michelin-starred chef in Korean cuisine. Hooni still visits Mr. Hwang at least once a year to continue learning this naturalistic approach. Calling Mr. Hwang seung seng nim, or his teacher, Hooni credits Mr. Hwang for inspiring his philosophies in his cooking and how he approaches every aspect of his life.

When I visited Mr. Hwang's operation in Jeju, I found myself in awe of what he had built. With the sound of the ocean crashing nearby, I watched as his rosy-cheeked grandchildren roamed through the beautiful gardens, made all the more lush from Jeju's clean water and fresh air. I entered the restaurant and tearoom, which were decorated like a museum commemorating the wisdom of Korea's past. The walls were adorned with Korean folklore paintings, beautifully hand-painted Korean ceramics, and medicinal roots like red ginseng and doraji (balloon flower) preserved in large liquid structures. I immediately felt like I was in a cocoon of detoxification and healing.

"How did you become so interested in Korea's old traditions?" asked Mr. Hwang. It was a question that I would receive time and time again on my travels, as people were surprised that someone from a newer generation would still be interested in Korea's past. Mr. Hwang and I sat and talked over a cup of tea. He seemed happy to discover the parallels in our health journeys. Despite our outward differences, we had each taken ownership of our health and learned how to heal naturally by first eating whole foods and being closer to nature. We had also discovered a similar silver lining to our health crises: Out of our unfortunate experiences emerged a new philosophy for living well. Although we had just met, we immediately bonded over our shared commitment to self-care and a food as medicine approach to wellness. I could not have been more thrilled when Mr. Hwang asked me to come back to visit him in Jeju again.

The work of the Hwang family, in collaboration with local producers like the haenyeo, has created a sustainable ecosystem in Jeju that showcases the best of what traditional eating has to offer. By using what the land can provide, taking only what is needed, and preparing meals with natural ingredients in their peak nutrient state, they remind us of how we can heal and nourish our bodies, while doing all of this sustainably.

Seaweed: The nutritional jewel of the sea

In the ocean's depths, haenyeo tend to a rich and hidden aquatic forest of seaweed. These seaweeds are the counterparts to the trees and plants on land, using solar energy to absorb CO_2, much like trees do, and to feed life within the ocean. Although seaweed can be as small as a one-celled phytoplankton, they can also grow in tangled systems as large as

150 feet long. Though often overlooked, they are an abundant, sustainable, and highly nutritious natural resource. Responsible for half of all oxygen production on Earth, these plants contain many minerals and nutrients that they absorb from their seawater bath.

Seaweeds are a part of the daily diets of centenarians throughout Asia, and they form the core of the haenyeo diet. Scientists have only just begun to discover their health benefits, which are manifold. They are protein-rich, they contain soluble fiber (which aids digestion), and they have omega-3 healthy fats. They have been linked to improving insulin resistance; suppressing weight gain; blocking cancer cell growth; lowering cholesterol, blood pressure, heart disease risk, and thyroid diseases; and increasing mental clarity. Eating just two tablespoons of miyeok (brown algae or wakame), for example, will give you 28 percent of the recommended daily requirement for iodine, manganese, folate, sodium, magnesium, calcium, iron, copper, phosphorus, and vitamins A, C, E,

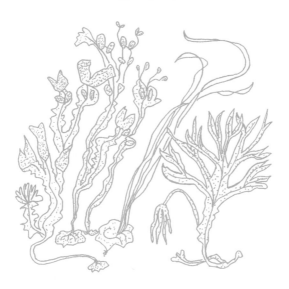

and K. Seaweeds are also touted to reduce cellulite and water retention, eliminate toxins from the body, and to have anti-inflammatory and anti-aging effects on the skin.

In Japan and Korea, miyeok (brown algae or wakame) and nori (red or black algae, used for sushi) comprise 75 percent of the national sea vegetable consumption. However, there are a variety of other sea vegetables to try that are highly nutritious and will bring a delicious umami flavor to your dishes:

- **Brown algae:** miyeok (or wakame), kombu, mozuku
- **Red algae and black algae:** nori, dulse
- **Green algae:** sea grapes, sea lettuce
- **Blue-green algae:** spirulina, chlorella

In Asia, seaweeds are most commonly sold in stores in dried form, to be rehydrated before cooking. There are so many ways to use them in your kitchen: incorporated in sushi rolls or sushi "burritos"; boiled in broth for a mild flavor; dusted in powdered form on soups, salads, or other dishes; as a snack in the form of crispy toasted sheets; or seasoned on their own as a side dish. There is even a type of low-calorie, zero-carb gluten-free noodle made from kelp, which is a seaweed. These thin, translucent noodles easily absorb the flavors of a dish and can be used as a substitute for traditional noodles in stir-fried or "ramen" dishes.

Each of the seaweed varieties has its strengths and unique flavors. Red dulse, when stir-fried, has a savory "bacon" taste. Mozuku, from centenarian-filled Okinawa, is typically served in a tasty, slippery side dish seasoned with vinegar; it has the highest levels of fucoidan (a polysaccharide present mainly in brown seaweed), linked to anti-cancer activities. Sea grapes from Okinawa, which look like miniature versions of their namesake and a favorite with my son, burst with a unique umami flavor. Kombu, the chewiest and thickest of the group, has the highest level of iodine, approximately ninety-five times that of nori, and contains an enzyme that helps to make beans more digestible (and less gas-producing) by breaking down their sugars; it is also a key ingredient for many stocks in Asia. Nori and sea lettuce provide high levels of bioavailable iron. In the freshwater class, spirulina and chlorella are popular powdered plant protein and vitamin B supplements to dust on smoothies and meals.

Miyeokguk (seaweed soup), Korean birthday soup

Like most other Korean babies, my first experience with seaweed was in the form of miyeokguk, a broth of nourishing brown seaweed (otherwise known as brown algae or wakame), at my baek-il, or one-hundredth-day celebration, a milestone tradition dating back to the eighteenth century that originated when the survival rate for babies was low. Traditionally, this was the first time the baby and mother were taken outside, and it was considered a sign that both mother and little one would live to see the first year post-delivery. Korean folklore tells how my ancestors noticed that whales ate seaweed to recover after giving birth. Seaweed was then served to women during postpartum care, and its detoxifying function made it ideal for their recovery.

When I became a mother, I used this traditional Korean soup as part of a regimen to recover the nutrients I lost while delivering my two babies, as well as to help me recover so I could produce quality milk to breastfeed them for their first year of life. Since then, I have made miyeokguk frequently at home, as many Koreans do. Miyeokguk is called birthday soup because it is a reminder of the day that your parents gave you life, and you have Korean birthday soup as a way of showing respect and giving thanks to your elders.

INGREDIENTS

1-square-inch piece dried miyeok (brown algae or wakame)

1 teaspoon toasted sesame oil

2 teaspoons minced garlic

1 ounce grass-fed beef brisket, cut into small pieces (optional)

¾ cup stock, such as chicken or vegetable

1 tablespoon gukganjang (Korean soup soy sauce) or other naturally brewed soy sauce

Dried mustard powder (optional)

METHOD

1. In a large bowl filled with room-temperature filtered water, soak the dried miyeok for 10 minutes. Remove the seaweed from the water and use kitchen scissors to cut it into bite-sized pieces. Reserve the soaking water for cooking, as it is highly nutritious.

2. Heat the sesame oil with the garlic in a large pan over medium-high heat. If using, lightly cook the beef in the sesame oil for 2 minutes, or until browned. Then add the seaweed.

3. Add the stock and ½ cup of the seaweed soaking water, increase the heat to high to bring it to a boil, then reduce the heat to maintain a low simmer. Simmer uncovered for 20 minutes, or until the meat is tender and the broth is "milky."

4. Remove from the heat. Sprinkle with dried mustard powder, if using.

Sumbisori: The haenyeo's healing breath

The haenyeo are prime examples of a population that coexists with nature and uses natural means to thrive. Without diving equipment, they rely on their bodies' ability to draw in a supply of air for each dive, even as they age. To do this safely, these women practice an ancient and simple breathing technique, passed down through generations, that allows them to build up their lung capacity and physical strength against the dangers of their repeated dives. This breathing technique, called sumbisori, helps the divers sustain prolonged dives through rhythmic inhalations and whistling exhalations.

Sumbisori has also become an essential aspect of the haenyeo's ability to survive and thrive as a community. Through sumbisori, the haenyeo communicate and keep track of one another while in the water. Back on land, their cemented bond carries through to sharing responsibilities and mutual aid through pregnancies, illnesses, and crises. Haenyeo researcher Cha Hyek-young suggests that the sounds of sumbisori act as "a nonverbal transmitter of memory, of resistance, of rising above the circumstances." The act of diving itself would also seem to support mental health in that it involves the cultivation of mindfulness, purpose, and engagement and promotes a connection to nature. Some women of younger generations are leaving modern lives to learn how to live like the haenyeo. For them, free diving into the cold waters every day is a way to combat depression and keep strong, all while making a living.

When we breathe, we take in oxygen, a resource that is vital for sustaining life. While breathing is a natural process, many might be surprised to learn that there is a right and a wrong way to breathe. Proper breathing starts with inhaling through the nose and exhaling out through the mouth. Practicing slow, mindful, deep belly breathing, rather than taking quick shallow breaths, is also important. Deep belly breathing involves allowing enough time to enable air to fill your lungs and chest cavity and expand your belly while contracting and moving your diaphragm downward. Breathing in this way, through the nose, allows for more oxygen to get to active tissues. It also allows the cilia, the tiny hairs in the nostrils, to filter out toxins and allergens from the air, preventing them from entering the body and causing illness, while also warming and humidifying the air so that it is not too cold or dry when it enters the lungs.

After discovering sumbisori, I began to think about my own breathing and made a concerted effort to be more intentional about it. I began cultivating a daily yoga practice that reminded me to return to my breath and to synchronize my movements with my breathing. By implementing more intentional breathing and learning more about it, I am now more conscious of employing its benefits. Breathing mindfully has also enabled me to boost my athletic performance, and it is a technique that I use to immediately relax in real time wherever I am, even when I'm just standing in line somewhere. Some of my yoga classes combine light weight training where I employ these breathing techniques. I have learned that the golden rule of lifting weights is to exhale on exertion while making controlled movements. So, for example, for a squat, you would inhale slowly on your way down, then exhale on your way up. For a curl, you would exhale when you lift the weight and inhale as you lower it slowly back down.

Whatever form of exercise you choose, if you don't breathe properly, you won't get enough oxygen, then you'll tire quickly, and you won't be able to achieve as much from your workouts. Since paying more attention to my breathing, my workouts have become a lot more efficient and I have become much stronger. In the past, I hadn't taken advantage of my body's natural mechanisms to help me thrive through efficient oxygen intake. Now, I like to think of myself taking sips of air throughout my workouts and throughout the day, as I do with water or other fluids.

When we focus on proper breathing form, we will also reap the benefits of better sleep and digestion, improved immune response, and more concentration and focus. Better breathing also benefits the parasympathetic nervous system, which opposes our fight-or-flight response, enabling us to stay calm and reduce stress.

I have experienced incredible benefits by being more intentional with my breath and practicing the following breathing exercises, which are recommended by the American Lung Association.[1]

Pursed lip breathing

1. Inhale slowly for 2 seconds through the nose, keeping the mouth closed
2. Pucker or purse the lips, as if whistling or blowing out a candle, exhaling slowly for 4 seconds
3. Repeat

Belly, or diaphragmatic, breathing

1. Follow steps above for pursed lip breathing while placing both hands on the belly
2. Feel the belly rise and fall with each breath

Hydration Culture

"Drink your tea slowly and reverently, as if it is the axis on which the world earth revolves—slowly, evenly, without rushing toward the future. Live the actual moment. Only this moment is life."[1]

—Thich Nhat Hanh, *Vietnamese monastic and peace activist*

One of my favorite experiences in Korea was sitting down with Mr. Hwang in Jeju to share a tea he made with his own personal mix of herbs, a tea he drank every day instead of water. After enjoying a delicious dinner prepared by his family, we gathered for this special tea. It was his way of inviting more intimate conversation in a relaxed setting following our meal, a shared communal experience for our collective well-being, with tea that warmed our hearts and our bellies.

Mr. Hwang's tea was made of organic ingredients including goji berry, red ginseng, ginger, and balloon flower, a bouquet he extensively researched to bring energy and vitality to the body. As we sat together in a simple room in his home, surrounded by his piles of books, I realized that this wasn't like one of the elaborate tea ceremonies one might imagine from a movie. For him, offering this tea was his way of nurturing and sharing a wholesome experience. He shared the belief underlying Korea's age-old national foundations that food is healing; food is medicine; food is love. Tea-drinking cultures across Asia—like Hong Kong, Japan, China, and Singapore—share this wellness philosophy in their histories, contributing to their longevity rates.

Koreans who subscribe to the traditional ways drink tea copiously, like water, especially the herbal, non-caffeinated varieties, and will even have their teas to go in a reusable bottle to experience their benefits throughout the day. Most notably, these teas contain polyphenols, or antioxidants, which diminish the damaging and aging effects of free radicals in the body. Throughout Asia, tea is ubiquitous. In the office, tea service is offered to employees right at their desks. Vending machines and convenience stores offer a wide range of unsweetened tea brands wherever you walk. And there is science behind drinking so much tea.

Researchers have found that the key to unlocking the health benefits of tea is quantity; they recommend drinking two or three or more cups daily.[2]

The idea that humans should hydrate and drink a constant supply of fluids for optimal health goes back centuries. **Just as the ocean needs constant replenishment from rainfall and rivers to supply lost water for life underneath to thrive, our bodies, too, require a constant replenishment of fluids, not only for keeping our cells alive but for having them function properly.** Whenever I feel the need for a reset after a period of unhealthy habits, the first step I take is to hydrate with fluids based on traditional Korean methods. I eat fruits and vegetables with a high water content, like watermelon or cucumber. I make it a point to consume broths, guk (Korean soups), water, teas, and electrolytes from salt. These are all hydration techniques that Koreans use to easily bring the body back to balance.

Our brains, muscles, blood, and other internal organs are made up of 75 to 85 percent water. Water moves nutrients and oxygen through the body, boosts our energy and alertness, and helps us to curb cravings. Water is such an essential nutrient that we can only survive without it for about three days. Without sufficient water, you may be surprised at just how significantly your overall functioning is depleted. When we are dehydrated, our heads begin to ache, we can't think at our peak levels, we can't run as fast, our skin dries up, and we aren't as flexible. Additionally, our kidneys need water to help us flush out our systems so that our bodies are not bogged down with waste, mucus, and toxins. And when we lose an estimated 1.5 to 3 liters of our bodily water daily through activities like breathing, sweating, even sleeping, we need to replace it. But we can stay hydrated by drinking more herbal teas, which flavor and add antioxidants to our water, making it easier, and more flavorful, to take in our fluids every day.

We also drink our tea warm or hot for health reasons. Drinking hot water or tea after a meal emulsifies fats, which aids digestion. It also increases blood flow and dilates blood vessels in the gut, which kick-starts the digestive system, especially when taken in the morning on an empty stomach. In Asia, locals tend to carry around thermoses filled with hot water for this reason. But not too hot; research suggests that water over 140°F may not be healthy for you and will destroy beneficial compounds in the tea.[3]

The most popular detoxifying tea drink in Korea

Green tea and its whole-leaf pulverized version, matcha (which I now drink often for its fat-burning, powerful antioxidants), are beloved around the world. But the most popular tea drink in Korea is boricha, or roasted barley tea, which is non-caffeinated and, therefore, can be drunk all day without affecting your sleep. Technically a tisane, a plant-derived drink, rather than tea derived from tea leaves, boricha has a nutty and mild flavor and is known for its detoxifying effects. Rich in antioxidants, the tea provides numerous health benefits, including curbing cravings, regulating blood sugar, aiding in digestion, and acting as a natural antacid that helps relieve heartburn and acid reflux.

This two-ingredient tea, made with barley grains and water, is healthy and delicious, and it can be brewed at home in minutes to be enjoyed either hot or cold, and served all year long. I grew up drinking boricha instead of water at meals in my Korean American household, unaware of its health benefits until I rediscovered this tradition on my health journey. When I drink more boricha, I feel light, clear, and energized. When I fall off track with my health goals, my first step to get back is to begin each day drinking at least two liters of boricha or water.

Preparing boricha to incorporate into your daily wellness routine is simple. Boil eight cups of water in a medium pot, then add three table-spoons of roasted barley grains, boiling for another five minutes. Or do as I do and buy the tea bags online and steep them for ten minutes to ensure that you are releasing the beneficial plant compounds into the drink, and refrigerate. Even at cold temperatures, the tea will still provide the same antioxidant and nutritional benefits. I also like to occasionally switch in two delicious substitutes: memil-cha (tea made with roasted buckwheat grains) or oksusu-cha (tea made with roasted corn or corn silk).

Jjimjilbang: Traditional Bathhouses

"The sauna is a poor man's pharmacy."

—*Finnish saying*

"The way to health is to have an aromatic bath and a scented massage every day."

—*Hippocrates*

A gaggle of elderly women don't bat an eye as I enter, barefaced and nude, into the first private room of a jjimjilbang, a traditional Korean spa. Bodies of all shapes and sizes come together in this misty bathhouse haze; some of us wrinkled, some smooth. We were all flesh and bones together, sharing in a moment of quiet intimacy, bonding in the purity of our humanness, and democratized without the obvious demarcations of our stations in life. In a jjimjilbang, guests must be comfortable exposing themselves in their most vulnerable state, without the armor and protection of their worldly disguises, shedding their clothes, shoes, jewelry, and bags, even their makeup.

I had once, long ago, visited a jjimjilbang in Korea as a child visiting relatives, but this was my first visit as an adult. I intended to go in for the whole experience. Upon paying the $8 admission, I was given a small locker, two tea towel–sized bath cloths, a plain cotton pajama shorts set, and unlimited access to revel in this private world for the day. I could even spend the night and purchase from a menu of snacks if I paid a little more. It seemed like a small price to pay for a break from the stresses of the outside world, a chance for ablution, to wash my worries away.

After storing my belongings under lock and key, I entered the first communal room, a steamy, white-tiled, open space with low vanity stations, each replete with a personal wall mirror and a tiny stool to sit on while using the shower head and soap to wash. To be allowed to enter the shared baths in the next room, each guest had to first wash off outside dirt and grime in this anteroom. The experience was like entering some sort of temple, then emerging reinvigorated with a cleansed body and a meditative state of mind.

Next, I entered the bathing room and dunked myself in and out of an assortment of hot and icy pools alongside a network of steam rooms of varying temperatures, experimenting with their various effects. My skin prepped, the outer layer loosened by the soak, I opted for a professional Korean scrub and massage, lying on a table at the back of the bathhouse. An older woman, an ahjumma, appeared in a black bathing suit. For an hour, she used thin exfoliating mitts to vigorously scrub the front and back of my body, removing the ddeh, or dead skin, in a vigorous exfoliation exercise that had no comparison. She created a foam by wringing a simple cotton cloth covered with liquid soap and spread this carefully all over my body, covering me in a delightful bubble bath before gently dousing me with buckets of warm water to wash my old skin away. Then she stretched my limbs and massaged my joints with oil.

I returned to the locker room to change into my pajama-like attire before entering to join the family-style common rooms where similarly dressed men, women, children, and young couples sat relaxing and socializing. People stretched out in all corners of these rooms, lying down to rest and sleep on the heated floors, walking back and forth from the connecting dry kiln saunas made of jade and salt. Like merpeople, we had emerged from our bathing pools to luxuriate on the warm shores of this man-made beach, wrapped in the warm comfort that we are all in this together.

Slicked, scraped, and scrubbed, my skin had never felt so silky smooth, with a glow that I had never been able to achieve before at home. I felt as relaxed as I had never been. And I wondered why I didn't do this more often.

Bathing cures for all in Korea

Ritual bathing has existed for centuries as a self-care practice in numerous cultures. In sixth-century Japan, influenced by Buddhist purification practices, hot springs known as onsens were built with the aim of ritual bathing, or to clean the body and spirit and improve overall health. The ancient Greeks built bathing facilities to cure disease; the Romans elaborated on this with formidable multiroom bathhouses called thermae, which featured dry and wet heat treatments for releasing tension and were seen as places for meditation and self-reflection. Communal bathhouses in ancient cultures tended to be accessible to all members of the community. In modern society, spa treatments are for the most part only available to those who can afford the price tag.

Korea's jjimjilbangs are the exception to this rule. **Open to the general public, jjimjilbangs are a unique feature of the modern spa landscape thanks to their affordability and "wellness for everyone" approach.** In Korea, children enter with adults, establishing the importance of self-care rituals early on in life. While the bathing areas are separated by gender, jjimjilbangs invite social bonding in mixed-age groups in shared, co-ed spaces. It is common for families to go together, couples to go for dates, and friends to go together to socialize. With their 24/7 rest zones, jjimjilbangs even serve as crash pads for some people after a night out. The casual and open nature of jjimjilbangs means that Koreans from all walks of life have access to a rich toolbox of self-care methods while spending time in a body-positive environment where everyone feels comfortable in their own skin.

The healing elements of a jjimjilbang

Jjimjilbangs offer a more approachable version of the restorative rituals once practiced by dynastic kings and queens of Korea. These ancient healing applications included heat and cold therapy, massage, and deep body exfoliation. Jjimjilbang, which literally means "heating room," exemplifies how heat is one of Korea's earliest healing traditions.

Heat therapy in Korea dates back to 5000 BCE during the Neolithic

Age, starting with early ondols, or heated floors, which are prevalent in jjimjilbangs. Ondols were originally constructed to provide an efficient system to keep homes warm. They manipulated the flow of smoke horizontally from fireplaces across underfloor ducts, allowing fire from the kitchen to simultaneously enable cooking and home heating, much different from the Western way of sourcing heat directly from the fire. The ondol system made the floor foundations uninhabitable for rats and bugs, keeping the homes clean and free of pests. It also allowed air inside a room to circulate naturally due to the laws of thermodynamics—hot air heated by the floor traveled upward, and the cold air was drawn downward. Many health benefits also came with ondols. The heat of the floors increases blood circulation in the legs, back, and ankles, which is helpful for arthritis. Ondols also prevent the circulation of dust particles that can cause allergies or sickness with forced air systems. Ondols made such an impression on the architect Frank Lloyd Wright during his time in Korea that he built one in his own home and employed this system in some of his buildings. Most families in Korea slept directly on these heated floors before high-rise apartments and Western-style beds arrived.

Inside a jjimjilbang, heat therapy is also provided through hot baths, which improve blood flow and make the blood more oxygenated by allowing one to breathe slowly and more deeply, particularly when taking in steam. The hot baths also relieve muscle tension, reduce nasal congestion, improve sleep, promote skin health, calm the nervous system, improve mood, and reduce anxiety and stress levels in the body.

Then there are the hot saunas, which promote a wide range of health benefits: anti-aging, detoxification, increased metabolism, weight loss, increased blood circulation, pain reduction, skin rejuvenation, improved cardiovascular function, improved immune function, improved sleep, stress management, and relaxation. Those made of salt in the jjimjilbangs provide halotherapy, or salt therapy, in which breathing in air with tiny salt particles improves breathing and is an alternative treatment for lung problems such as asthma, bronchitis, and coughing. Those made of jade are thought to improve the health of the kidneys, respiratory system, heart, liver, spleen, and glandular system. Saunas at jjimjilbangs come in the form of hot steam rooms and those that provide infrared heat, which has been shown to help lower inflammation levels and improve skin tone by delivering more oxygen and nutrients to the skin through increased circulation.

At the jjimjilbang, the hot saunas and hot baths are used in conjunction with the cold treatments—cold rooms and icy cold baths. These combined therapies have been shown to help increase metabolism, reduce inflammation and swelling, relieve sore muscles, aid exercise recovery, support immunity, and improve mental health, stress, and mood by reducing cortisol levels. Research has shown that daily cold showers at 20 degrees can be used as a proxy for cold treatments and are a potential treatment for depression.[1] Additionally, using a sauna five to fifteen times per month is directly associated with higher mental well-being scores compared to those who used the sauna less frequently.[2]

Massage and body exfoliation treatments at jjimjilbangs have proven benefits as well. Massage improves circulation, decreases muscle stiffness and joint inflammation, improves quality of sleep, speeds recovery between workouts, improves flexibility, and strengthens immune response. Body exfoliation increases circulation, boosts the skin's radiance, and aids cell turnover, making the skin look more glowing. Regular exfoliation can also help prevent clogged pores, resulting in fewer breakouts. The Korean version of vigorous body exfoliation has no comparison to any other culture, producing incredible skin results.

My first adult visit to a jjimjilbang in Korea was very different from what I remembered from my childhood days when I was rushed by the adults accompanying me to clean and finish up quickly. This time, I basked in the experience, taking the time to explore and playfully experiment with the extensive range of wellness offerings. It was like being in an amusement park for wellness. With so much on offer at such a reasonable price, I wished I lived near one back home to soak, sweat, exfoliate, and purify every day. I have taught my children the benefits of bath rituals, and now they choose to draw their own baths to relax, soak, and melt away their worries from their long school days.

Light stretching is a national pastime

Stretching was incorporated into my massage and body exfoliation in the jjimjilbang, but stretching in Korea is not limited to spas. It is common to see people in Korea stretching at random intervals during the day, whether against a tree, on a bench, or on an airplane. Stretching is such an accepted behavior in Korea that no one looks twice if they notice someone on the street stopping to stretch. Koreans of all ages love to stretch.

During COVID-19, the Korean government, in collaboration with the Korean Sport & Olympic Committee, released a YouTube video featuring national athletes reintroducing traditional gymnastics stretches. This was meant to encourage citizens to stay active and healthy during social distancing. These included arm and neck circles, knee bends, and various stretches for sides, chest, back, abs, and torso. Stretching keeps the muscles flexible, strong, and healthy. Today, as we spend an increasing number of sedentary hours in front of computer screens and scrolling through our phones, regular stretching is more important than ever. If we don't make the time to stretch, we lose flexibility and our muscles shorten and become tight, unable to fully function when called upon for physical activity. Athletes who know the importance of stretching to prepare for exercise or competition and to prevent injuries maintain a supple fascia. This connective tissue surrounds and holds bone, muscle, nerves, blood vessels, and organs in place. Stress to a particular part of the body from repeated exercise such as daily running will cause the fascia to tighten, causing pain and possible injury. Stretching resolves this and benefits us by increasing blood flow, relieving stress, improving mood, preventing injury, easing joint and muscle pain, and increasing flexibility and athletic performance. I decided to incorporate stretching at home as part of my wellness routine, even while taking periods of rest away from my computer. I will get up to take opposite movements from my usual computer stance, like opening my arms wide or walking around to keep my body flexible and working better longer.

The importance of slowing down

One evening while doing some home organizing, I rediscovered one of my kids' old picture books, *A Bear and His Boy* by Sean Bryan and Tom Murphy. I was dumbstruck by how this children's book, which I had read many times when my children were smaller, summarized my tendency for modern-day busyness. The bear in the story, Mack, spends his day stressed out and "running around like a maniac" on a schedule that is "totally packed," filled with quarterback duties, collecting an award, learning French, and so on, until the boy, Zack, rings the alarm bells to force Mack to stop for a moment to relax, appreciate the beauty of the little things, and "smell the lilacs."

We undervalue the importance of rest, but slowing down and giving our bodies and minds time to recover and return to homeostasis during busy times is essential to our health. Otherwise, we expose ourselves to the adverse physiological effects of chronic stress. Stress is a part of life, and small or moderate amounts of stress can benefit the body: taking a cold plunge bath or shower at the jjimjilbang; powering through a tough workout; rising to the challenge of a leadership position at work. However, when unmanaged stress overwhelms us, in the form of a toxic relationship, grief over the death of a loved one, or unrelenting pressure at work, it threatens to become chronic and can have damaging physical and mental health effects. Chronic stress is believed by many experts, including the World Health Organization and the American Psychological Association, to be the top health epidemic of our modern world. It is estimated that 75 to 90 percent of all doctor visits are stress-related.[3]

When you encounter a perceived threat, your brain's hypothalamus triggers an alarm system, prompting your adrenal glands to release a surge of hormones, including adrenaline and cortisol. These stress hormones flood the body, causing a fight-or-flight response, and can trigger gastrointestinal issues like mine. When stressors are constantly present, long-term activation of this stress-response system can lead to digestive problems, heart disease, impairment in memory and focus, depression, anxiety, headaches, sleep problems, and weight gain. In one study of a group of students during a stressful three-day exam period, their immunity decreased: they produced fewer NK cells, and their infection-fighting T-cells were less responsive. Excessive cortisol levels can also compromise the immune system by weakening the gut-immune barrier, specifically by lowering an antibody called IgA, which acts as a first line of protection in our digestive tract. When this happens, viruses are able to more readily invade through the lining of the intestinal tract.

Slowing down has positive effects on mindfulness too. When you take the time to pause, reflect, and identify areas of your life that need more attention, you will make better decisions, experience more gratitude, and even boost your creativity. In his book *The Things You Can See Only When You Slow Down*, Princeton-educated Korean Buddhist monk Haemin Sunim writes about how our fast-paced world can quickly become overwhelming. Even minor setbacks can seem catastrophic, making the more significant problems all the more devastating. "When you are so busy that you feel perpetually chased, when worrying thoughts circle your head, when the future seems dark and uncertain, when you are hurt by what someone has said, slow down, even if only for a moment. Bring all of your awareness into the present and take a deep breath."[4]

Taking the time to slow down periodically may not come naturally in our 24/7 digital world where we struggle to sit still or put away our phones. I know these things are challenges for me. But, as I discovered the hard way, it is critical to our health to switch off and take breaks. Although I had previously relied on stress to power through tasks, I came to realize that this unhealthy habit was taking a toll on me with real physiological consequences. Alternating cycles of activity with periods of rest is vital to keeping our bodies healthy—otherwise, we will burn out. Leading up to my emergency hospital visit, I was not prioritizing rest, and that was preventing my body from repairing everyday wear and tear. I needed to build purposeful breaks into my routine.

Bathhouse habits for transforming the body and the mind

Following my visit to the jjimjilbang, I brought home several practices and implemented them in my daily routine. The first was beginning each day whenever I could with a good sweat and detox with a hot yoga class. Then, in the evening, I began my newly found bath-care routine, taking nightly baths with a budget-friendly Epsom lavender salt and bubble bath mixture. This proved very effective at helping me to relax and get to sleep, soothing sore muscles, and leaving my body skin baby soft.

After the bath, the next part of my self-care routine was a nightly self-massage, starting from my feet and working up to my scalp, paying attention to every inch of my body and noticing any changes that might require medical care. I use my hands for this massage, along with new tools to promote circulation, fluid drainage, dead skin cell removal, and brighter skin: a dry brush for my body, a gua sha stone for gentle face and neck massage, then a little infrared electric wand. I purchased these budget-friendly bathcare tools along my travels across Asia but they are also easily found online.

The purpose of my self-massage is to encourage lymphatic drainage. This involves gently manipulating the lymph nodes in the neck, under the arms, and the groin to help drain the lymph, which carries waste products away from the tissues and back toward the heart. Lymphatic drainage relieves swelling in the body area that you are working on,

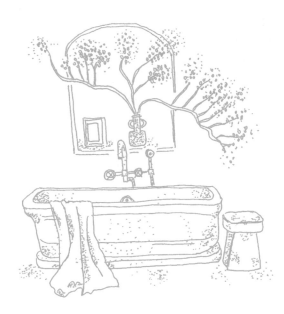

like your stomach or your face. It helps to drain excess water while also improving circulation and relaxing the body. Beyond self-massage, I was also encouraging lymphatic drainage through exercise, hot and cold showers, and increased fluid intake.

My skin-care routine has also changed. Previously, I used heavy body creams on my face, which I replaced with natural face oils, oil-based cleansers, balms, and serums as a daily part of my routine. I also try to be mindful of the quality of ingredients that my skin is being exposed to, finding as many nontoxic and eco-friendly products as possible. Before, I applied moisturizer twice a day—once in the morning after showering and once at night before bed. Now, I have started to carry a small bottle of lotion and some rose water mist, which I use to freshen my skin as needed throughout the day. With my skin health improved, I found that I did not necessarily need foundation, just a tiny dab of serum or facial oil on my cheeks and forehead. Happily, I began to see a glowing, dewy effect, and I credit it to feeding my skin health, both inside and out.

My father has always made it a point of gifting me—and later including my children—teas, healthy foods, face masks, and lotions, which, for a long time, I didn't link to my wellness. But now I understand that Koreans believe that nourishing your skin, and the fruits of that labor, is a visible sign of your health.

These practices, adapted from the bathhouses, now begin and end my days, and they are essential for helping me to slow down, take care of myself, and quiet my mind. I look forward to these moments and they help me to live each day with more calm and grace. I can barely remember what life was like before.

How to dry brush your body

- Take a dry brush tool and gently massage your skin using light pressure, moving in short, upward strokes

- Begin at the tops of your feet and work upward toward your ankles, calves, thighs, sides of the abdominal area, and buttocks. The idea is to always brush toward your heart
- When you reach your torso area, move in a circular clockwise motion to aid digestion
- Move to your chest, then your back, brushing downward toward your heart
- Finish with your hands, wrists, and the length of your arms with movements toward your heart
- Note: You will need a softer dry brush for your face

How to gua sha

Apply a facial oil, serum, or moisturizer before you start so that the gua sha tool glides on your skin.

- **Cheeks:** Place the flat, wide edge of the tool to the right of your mouth. Slowly move it upward past your cheekbone, applying gentle pressure, and stop right before you reach your ear. Repeat on the opposite side
- **Jawline:** Starting from the center of your chin, move the curved side of the tool along your jawline until you reach the base of your ear. Repeat on the opposite side
- **Forehead:** Starting from the top of your right eyebrow, gently drag the wide edge of the tool up to the top of your hairline. Repeat the motion starting from the middle of your eyebrows and above your left eyebrow
- **Eyes:** Starting just below the inner corner of your right eye, gently move the narrow side of the tool under your eye and toward your hairline. Repeat on the opposite side
- **Eyebrows:** Place the tool in the middle of your eyebrows and

sweep to the right until you reach your hairline. Repeat on the opposite side

- **Neck:** Starting from your right collarbone, sweep the wide side of the tool upward to your jawline while applying medium pressure, then repeat on the opposite side. Do each step twice before moving on to the next step
- **Throat:** Place the tool between your collarbones and lightly massage your throat by sweeping up to your chin. You can use the wide edge or one of the curved sides
- I always end a gua sha session with a quick self-massage using my bare hands to go a little deeper into my jawline, forehead, and cheeks. This extra step has significantly improved the bounce of my facial muscles and cleared water retention in my face

CARE

When ssukgat is nurtured with loving care, it can be cultivated into bountiful fields. With the right treatment, it will grow in abundance with bushy stems and gloriously haloed flowers, vibrant and well over a full and long life.

My Holistic Approach to Healing

"The doctor of the future will give no medicine, but will interest his patient in the care of the human frame, in diet and the cause and prevention of disease."

—Thomas Edison

There are two schools of medicine. One is Western, or "conventional" medicine, which many throughout the world use to reactively treat acute illness, disease, or health emergencies (as I did when I had my own hospital visit). The other is traditional Eastern medicine, which includes modalities like traditional Chinese medicine, and is based on the idea that we can use food and lifestyle changes to treat low-level illnesses like the common cold, and to prevent more serious, chronic illness.

Eastern medicine is practiced throughout Asia, where city streets are dotted with spice markets and herbal apothecaries selling treatments intended to address minor ailments such as coughs, colds, and digestive issues. Visiting an herbalist in Asia is a much more casual affair than making an appointment with a Western medical practitioner. Just walk in and mention your needs, and you will leave with a low-cost, nourishing mix of medicinal plant herbs and roots pummeled into a powder to be steeped in teas and soups. Throughout Asia, these two healthcare systems run in tandem and complement one another.

In Korea, healthcare starts well before going to the doctor, with functional foods and home cooking. In a traditional Korean home, it is common for family members to have a basic knowledge of home remedies, and recipes are passed down through generations to treat coughs, sore throats, or headaches, and to aid with recovery from childbirth, minor surgeries, and injuries. For immunity and respiratory support, one might add a small amount of a medicinal root like astragalus or ginseng to soups and broths, lending a sweet, earthy flavor. Dendrobium (orchid) root might also be steeped in tea for its purported neuroprotective and anti-inflammatory properties. When my son had a persistent cough, my friend Janice, a long-term former resident of Hong Kong, knew to prescribe monk fruit tea, telling me where to buy it in the local market. And healthy flavor layers, like ginger, star anise, mushrooms, and ferments, are all par for the course in a traditional Asian kitchen. This is the type of knowledge, along with a preventative approach to health, that is invaluable in our world filled with viral infections and chronic disease.

Throughout my health journey, I found myself increasingly drawn into a world filled with these traditional remedies. I began to immerse myself in studying these traditions, finding my Eastern-oriented coursework to be a fascinating complement to my Western-oriented coursework in holistic food and lifestyle. And because these traditional ways are by necessity and inherently environmentally friendly, finding a way to incorporate them into my routine fell in line with my values and how I wanted to live my life.

One of the most fascinating objects I came across on my travels was an item in the gift shop of the Temple of the Eight Immortals in Xi'an, China, outlining similar wellness principles to those practiced in Korea. It was a small octagonal wooden frame that held the image of a bagua trigram, which encapsulates various ancient Eastern life principles: the five elements of nature (water, wood, fire, earth, and metal), yin and yang (the two opposing energetic forces believed to exist within everything in nature and the universe), and the eight pillars of Taoism (a centuries-old healing system for preventative healthcare that includes exercise, balanced diet, herbology, massage, meditation, and acupuncture). I would later learn that the symbols depicted on the bagua all represented natural ways of clearing our internal pathways—from our energetic pathways to our nasal passageways to our circulatory systems to our bowels—in order to allow the body to be free to perform its functions.

The bagua is a powerful visual statement of how it is necessary for our health to rebalance when we are faced with the changes and pressures of life. Perhaps you don't buy into these traditional concepts, but in fact, many of the principles of the bagua are aligned with what we know logically to be true. **Every time we make a lifestyle decision—for example, how we eat or drink—we move our body and our mind toward balance or imbalance.** We can do things to clear our system, including breathwork, movement, consuming a healthy diet, and managing our stress. These activities allow us to have more energy to be our best selves in body and in mind.

Throughout my travels, I met others who, like me, had taken the next step to learn about lifestyle through an Eastern lens and belief system. Many of these people were doing so in an attempt to heal their own chronic health issues, which had not responded to conventional drug protocols. They were a cast of characters of all ages, each with their own health story. I connected with an eighty-five-year-old macrobiotic hippie who was a staunch vegan due to the politics around food; a nutrition expert for celebrities and power executives; a managing director from a popular New York City wellness center; a Taoist master; a Pilates studio owner; a tai chi master; a few Michelin-starred chefs; and a fascinating woman in her sixties named Nancy who was a former librarian at Columbia University and who over a decade had read a full library of health books donated by a wealthy patron. I also met doctors, business leaders, public health experts, and farmers who are working to meld new science with tradition. Then I joined the board of GrowNYC, an environmental nonprofit, which firmly believes that healthy food access is a basic human right. These individuals are pioneering a new frontier in health and well-being—one in which we live and eat sustainably, in harmony with the natural world, melding centuries-old well-being wisdom with new science.

My conversations with these fellow travelers led to many suggestions of new ways to improve my lifestyle. With each new discovery, I furiously scrawled and sketched what I learned in my notebooks. Each person I talked to had a slightly different approach to what was best for their body, which sometimes included vitamin supplements or different types of movement. But we all shared the common thread of using natural, plant-based ingredients, and striving for balance and moderation. We all also shared an openness to trying new things, and a curiosity to learn from the traditions of other cultures.

We discussed the importance of combining Western and Eastern medicine, the belief that many chronic illnesses are preventable and reversible with lifestyle changes, and the idea that we must understand the root causes of our illnesses and first try natural interventions before other medical solutions. My experiences on these trips also made me more aware and appreciative of the wisdom and vast array of health traditions from around the world. We are all bound by our human spirits. Our differences are often only skin deep, with our varying beliefs shaped by unique experiences and living environments. This was a lesson that opened my heart and mind to new perspectives.

Along the way, I realized then that my explorations had changed me in ways that extended far beyond healing my body. Now, I had endless questions for my parents about why certain things were important in Korean culture, and how things came to be. One day, they retold the story of how my grandfather went to a name specialist in Korea to choose the Hanja characters for Jungmin, my Korean name. My grandfather returned home to call us in Brooklyn. He had decided that my name would consist of the characters that meant "pure" and "intellect," or "pure mind." He was, after all, an educator. When I was growing up, I had desperately asked my parents to name me Samantha after seeing a celebrity on an American TV show. Jungmin was always my middle name, but I never used it, despite the thoughtfulness that I now understand came with its selection. As a child, sometimes I had wanted to eschew my ethnicity, the difference to my American friends that would draw attention and require a need to explain. But now I prefer to use my Korean name as my grandfather had named me. I want to continue connecting back to my cultural identity that had laid relatively hidden until now. These days, I try to notice more and ask deeper questions about my Korean origins. My curiosity has also led to finding connections in different cultures and prompted me to travel the world more.

My health reset

After my emergency hospital visit, I decided that it was important to connect with as many people as possible as I set out on my path to healing. On my quest to repair my broken digestive system, I spoke with doctors, nutritionists, wellness experts, and acquaintances who had dealt with similar issues. I listened to every podcast and read every book I could get my hands on. Through these conversations, I was shocked to discover many others out there who were quietly struggling with similar gut issues and who had accepted that this was just a part of life.

Most of the individuals facing similar health issues, and who did not know of the solutions I later discovered, assumed that their suffering was normal. The summer after my health issues began, I complemented what I was learning in Asia and booked an appointment with a functional medicine doctor in New York who had been highly recommended by a friend. Conventional medicine for the most part treats what is above the surface—symptoms and disease. Functional medicine, by contrast, attends to what is below the surface, at the root of the disease: environmental and lifestyle factors, including sleep and relaxation; physical activity; nutrition; stress; relationships; clean air; and water.

This functional doctor ordered a comprehensive blood panel, which included additional tests on my micronutrient levels, as well as a food sensitivity test. The reports were highly informative and surprising. My food sensitivity test showed that my body was not responding well during my illness to what I thought was a healthy breakfast of two to four eggs each morning. It also showed that string beans, of all things, were not compatible with my impaired digestive system. More extended bloodwork revealed that I was also deficient in vitamins D and B$_{12}$, which needed to be remedied by spending more time exposed to sunlight, eating more vitamin-rich foods, or taking vitamin supplements. Come to think of it, I did feel a bit queasy every day after breakfast, but I'd figured it was just the pre-meeting work buzz that was a normal start to my day. How many others out there were unknowingly eating too much of something that was actually working against them, or eating a nutrient-poor diet that wasn't properly fueling their bodies?

With the help of the functional doctor, I was put on a prescription range of vegan plant-based tinctures and powders to heal my gut, including glutamine powder, licorice root, and bone broth powder; probiotics to support the growth of healthy bacteria in my stomach; and gentian bitter root capsules to ease any bloating that might occur. My functional doctor also suggested a simpler diet of whole foods and that for a few weeks I take a break from the eggs and string beans, foods that I was not tolerating with my impaired gut, to give it a chance to heal.

During this period, I prepared gentle, gut-healing recipes and broths (see the recipe for green papaya and fish soup, page 187) and pineapple and papaya, tropical fruits with digestive enzymes. These were healing methods that I learned from the keeper of traditional methods in my family. With families in Asia keeping to the traditional ways more steadfastly, these healing recipes tend to be preserved through adulthood. I began to truly understand that food was their love language and important culturally for them to show that they cared.

As I made these changes to allow my body to heal, I noticed a resetting of my palate. I found myself enjoying the natural sweetness of a simple piece of fruit and craving the taste and smells of rich broths simmering on the stovetop. My skin also became extremely clear. As time passed, I felt increasingly lighter and more energetic. I also started to feel much better physically. With my gut on the way to full recovery, my stomach pains after each meal had all but disappeared. After my gut healed, I'm happy to report that I am able to enjoy eggs and string beans again. I also try to focus more on eating whole foods. This is what worked best for me. But the search for what causes inflammation or sensitivity is highly personal. If you are looking for health solutions, I wholly recommend making changes in tandem with seeing a doctor. Your doctor can help you with tests for food sensitivities, to find vitamin deficiencies, and the like.

My period of recovery was a family affair. When a parent is down, the ties that bind your household can come loose. My friends and family members rose to the occasion, doing double duty with the kids so that I could rest. They also cared for me by making all sorts of traditional recipes that their elders had taught them, including slow-cooked broths that I would drink throughout the day, and dishes that incorporated fresh fruits and vegetables. The support from them and the food made with love helped beyond measure.

Outside of food, one of the most profound lessons that I experienced was learning how to take periods of slowing down. I understood now in observing the centenarians of Asia that there was no need to rush to accomplish my life goals. If I took care of my body, I would have more time than I previously thought to do them. Taking a break from the frantic whirlwind that had previously characterized my work life was also invaluable. I had gotten used to constant exhaustion, and my run-down body was begging for more frequent breaks. After some initial hesitation, I finally even started experimenting with short bursts of meditation like the Buddhist nuns do with the help of an app called Headspace, which guides you through momentary stillness with the voice of Andy Puddicombe, a former Buddhist monk.

For my friend Minh, who grew up with Chinese Buddhist parents and began following Korean Buddhist teachings as a student at Yale and now, while living as a busy executive in Hong Kong, meditation is a way of life, and he gave me pointers on how to start. He advised me that meditation is three parts of body, breath, and mind. First, sit up straight while trying to relax every cell in your body, including your face, shoulders, and chest. He finds that keeping the eyes half open resting on the ground helpful to stay awake in the moment. Then he goes about breathing as discussed on page 144. He is a wonderful example of how wellness traditions from the past can be brought forward successfully as a busy professional in the modern world. He attributes his practice to his successes in life, staying calm in moments of crisis and having purpose.

My full recovery with natural methods led me to wonder: Why weren't there more people recommending these natural first steps? I felt like I'd made an incredible discovery that altered myself in such a radical way, and I wanted others to share in it too.

My experimentations taught me that food plays one of the biggest—if not *the* biggest—role in the state of our personal health. The food we eat provides our body's cells the instructions to function and the raw materials it needs to function properly. I also know that food needs to work in conjunction with things like daily movement and stress management. Without healthy inputs, our metabolic processes break down and our health declines, as had happened to me. I had shed my old skin, taken Neo's red pill, and could never look back to the way I used to live.

What really makes us sick

Nineteenth-century French chemist Louis Pasteur devised the germ theory—the idea that germs cause disease, which paved the way for medical interventions like the use of antibiotics. But Pasteur had a friend and colleague, physiologist Claude Bernard, who theorized that germs weren't making us directly sick. Rather, Bernard believed that the cause of illness was the resiliency of the body's terrain. Terrain-based treatment is a natural approach that taps into the power of nutrition and lifestyle changes to support optimal health and well-being, and it is discussed extensively in the international bestseller *Anticancer,*[1] written by French scientist and physician David Servan-Schreiber. Bernard believed that the terrain was more important than germ theory in understanding what really makes us sick and that our bodies even harbored microorganisms—the microbiome, which we now know is more important for health than ever. The terrain theory holds that when we are exposed to germs, we become ill if our defenses are weakened by immune deficiencies or toxicities; we do not get sick just by the exposure to the germs themselves.

Modern medicine focuses on eliminating the symptoms, rather than treating the terrain, the soil of our bodies. But this terrain is an essential aspect of medical intervention throughout Asia, where complementary treatment can simultaneously encourage our body's natural defenses against disease. Unlike germ theory, terrain theory explains why some people get sick, while others, exposed to the same pathogens, do not. **By embracing terrain theory, we can orient ourselves toward remedying the weaknesses in our terrains to prepare our bodies for what they need to defend against disease.** Incorporating a terrain approach means that you are taking a longer-term perspective to improving your health—one that is natural and preventative, and that will serve you better in the long run.

Thinking back to the years preceding my emergency hospital visit, I now recognize the early warning signs: chronic stress, small stomach pains, poor sleep, and fatigue. The ongoing stress that my body was under was depleting my microbiome, my gut bacteria, and my stomach lining, leading to inflammation in my gut. When stress is chronic, it is medically critical to take a break—even a small one—in that hyperactive cycle to get your body back to homeostasis so that it is functioning normally. **Chronic stress is prevalent in today's culture, and it not only disrupts the microbiome but it wreaks havoc on every system in the body—the immune, digestive, reproductive, and circulatory systems—in addition to contributing to premature aging (a sign that our cells are breaking down at a faster than normal rate).**

Before my health crisis, I was arrogant enough to think that I was above getting truly sick, as I was exercising regularly and eating (mostly) healthy foods. I thought that all the stress I was under was good. It kept me going, and stress can be good in *temporary* doses. But my stress was chronic, and I powered through, continually ignoring the signs that my health was being compromised. Ironically, coming from a family of doctors, I didn't understand the importance of practicing self-care *before* my health was in crisis. Beyond going to the doctor for checkups, exercising, and eating a somewhat healthy diet, I was unaware of how to detect signs of imbalance in my system.

Inflammation is an age-old word that comes from the Latin *inflammare*, meaning to ignite or burn. Inflammation isn't a big deal if it lasts for a few days, like swelling from a finger prick. After all, it is the immune system's normal response to an infection or injury. But if you suffer from chronic inflammatory pain that persists for months or years, it likely indicates a deeper problem brewing. Low-level inflammation may first appear in mild forms such as headache; fatigue; poor memory and brain function; poor vision; shortness of breath; bloating; excess weight; frequent bruising or bruises that take a long time to heal; darkening or thickening of the skin; restless sleep; weak, sore muscles; dental cavities; fallen feet arches; and even premature wrinkles. These seemingly benign symptoms could be early signs of more advanced inflammation (e.g., the onset of heart disease) to come if they go unaddressed.

Two years after publishing his bestseller *Anticancer*, author David Servan-Schreiber discovered through numerous conversations and new research that the mind-body connection was critical enough to warrant a second, revised edition of his bestseller, with an added chapter called "The Anticancer Mind." In it he argues that when negative feelings, like tensions and worries, are left unattended, becoming chronic and/or worsening, they contribute to the inflammatory process that can help cancer—and other diseases—to grow.

The mind-body connection is now well-documented in scientific studies, but it never occurred to me, before that my stress was not only chronic but that it was having negative physical effects on my body. As physician Gabor Maté explores in his book *When the Body Says No*,[2] the hidden cost of stress is a negative impact on our immune system. Maté explains that disease is the body's way of saying "no" to what the mind cannot or will not acknowledge, for our emotions are electrical, chemical, and hormonal discharges from the nervous system, which influence major organs and our immune system. In *The Body Keeps the Score*,[3] Bessel van der Kolk explains how negative memories, particularly the stress from trauma, change how the brain regulates bodily functions. According to van der Kolk, "Neuroscience research shows that the only way we can change the way we feel is by becoming aware of our inner experience and learning to befriend what is going on inside ourselves."

What it means to heal

As with functional medicine, from a traditional medicine perspective, prevention is the best form of healthcare. Many in the Western world, myself included, have failed to take this approach, only paying attention to self-care after the onset of a health crisis. However, it's never too late, or too early (as young Korean children show us) to take a proactive, preventive approach to managing our health through self-awareness and early detection and intervention. If we commit to living this way, it is possible to effectively wipe out the root causes for larger health problems down the road. And this isn't hard to do. **We can all make simple modifications to our nutrition and lifestyle routines to prevent chronic inflammatory conditions—a focus on natural foods, daily movement, exposure to the natural world, rest and stress management, and getting emotional support from relationships. The power to self-heal is in our own hands.**

I discovered that eliminating added refined sugar from my diet allowed me to feel my best physically and at my most energetic. I enjoyed savory and fermented soups more than the sweetened smoothies I was drinking, and gradually, the majority of my plant dishes became more savory too. I still eat eggs (and love them), along with string beans, but less frequently than I used to, and I find that I feel much better as a result.

Friends often ask me how long it took to "heal" after embarking on this new way of eating and living. Everyone's journey will be individualized and different, but for me, it took a total of two years to heal my body, mind, and spirit. While I felt better immediately after cutting a food item like refined sugar out of my diet, my overall transformation—from a workaholic who never cooked and barely slept, to a person who laughs more and spends time daily thinking about how to nourish herself and her loved ones—was much more gradual. I began to also extend the idea of what was nourishing from my physical body to the other aspects of my life—spending more time on what was feeding my spirit, including seeking authentic friendships and doing more of the things that brought me joy, like hiking, drawing, listening to music, and reading books.

According to Korean Buddhist monk Haemin Sunim, "Don't struggle to heal your wounds. Just pour time into your heart and wait. When your wounds are ready, they will heal on their own." One can never underestimate the healing power of time, and slowing down is part of this. And perhaps we are never fully "healed." Because healing is a lifelong journey for each of us, dealing with life's cycles of ups and downs.

The Three Treasures

At the center of the Korean flag is a red and blue circle, the taegeuk, which symbolizes cosmic balance, the constant interaction between the yin and the yang. Yin and yang originated as a Chinese philosophical concept, where opposite forces are seen as complementary, interconnected, and interdependent in the natural world, and how they may give rise to each other as they interrelate to one another. My Korean ancestors must have believed that humans exist inseparably between heaven (represented by the upper red section of the taegeuk, or yang) and earth (the lower blue section of the taegeuk, or yin) and that there is a mutual relationship between these three and a means to live in harmony.

The taegeuk represents the diametric opposites in the natural world around us—light and dark; hot and cold; fire and water; masculine and feminine. Traditional medicine is predicated on maintaining a balance between yin and yang in the body. When there is an imbalance, we get sick. There is an expectation that the body needs constant monitoring and resetting to get back to homeostasis. For example, when the body is too hot, we must cool it down. When we lose water and salt through sweating, we need to replenish these in our body. We must also eat seasonally and respect what the environment can offer to maintain balance.

Our minds, bodies, and spirits are in a constant state of flux, and we will always need to bring them back to balance. To keep that homeostatic balance, those who practice traditional Chinese medicine maintain the Three Treasures: jing (essence), qi (life force), and shen (spirit, mind-heart). There is an old analogy often used to explain these concepts through the image of a candle. Jing is the body of the candle, the wax and wick, the main structure and foundation of the Three Treasures, determined by your genetic inheritance and energy reserves. Qi is the flame, the source of light, and your vitality or daily energy. Shen is the light that radiates from the burning candle. When jing and qi are in abundance, shen is released. The Three Treasures describe the physiological functions of all living organisms and are the essential energies believed critical for human life to be sustained and to thrive. If you're not tending to the fire, it will die out. **We can expect that throughout our lives, our wellness levels will ebb and flow, and that we will periodically need to bring ourselves back to balance.** The ways that our mind, body, and spirit relate to our environment are interconnected and constantly changing, meaning we must monitor them and adapt accordingly to maintain balance. I am certainly not perfectly eating, cooking, or exercising all the time, but I know how to get back into balance when I get off track. There will never be a point where we are 100 percent "fixed"; we will always be perfectly imperfect works in progress, and to me, this is what living life is all about. I also know that when I experience a challenging period, I can focus on improving this aspect of my life force through the natural methods outlined in this book, and this work can only lead to a positive outcome.

Food and fluids for faster recovery

Prevention is key to a long, healthy life. But what happens when we inevitably catch something and get sick? The common cold can affect a single person up to eight times per year, with symptoms that include coughing, sore throat, runny nose, sneezing, headaches, body aches, fatigue, and fever. Colds are no fun, but they are a prime opportunity for using nutrient-dense foods and fluids to shorten our recovery period. At the start of a cold, if our body awareness of any oncoming symptoms is on the alert, only a few adjustments are required to reverse the illness early, including clearing congestion and phlegm. While the cold will still have to run its course, prompt treatment can reduce the duration of the illness and prevent symptoms from progressing.

According to Eastern medicine, a healthy organism will tend to correct its own minor imbalances if allowed to do so, just as the Korean Buddhist nuns taught me. The body has the ability to heal itself, provided it is given what it really needs. With minor ailments, the body will do its own natural clean-out and the illness will run its course, provided we stay hydrated to help flush toxins out. Many Eastern practitioners believe that Western over-the-counter medications that interfere with the body's self-healing ability can hinder this process. Cold medicines, for example, only serve to suppress symptoms like mucus, which should be expelled from the body.

In traditional Asian cuisine, food is not only prepared to be easily digestible, it is also discretely paired with digestive aids like fermented foods and condiments, probiotic-rich soups, gelatinous broths, fruit with digestive enzymes, and hydrating fluids at every meal.

These digestive aids also work well to treat the common cold. General rules of thumb for recovering from a cold include eating fewer solid foods; consuming lots of fluids (broths, water, watery porridges); and eating light, easily digestible foods like cooked greens in a bland state (e.g., avoiding sugar or high salt). A sample diet during cold recovery might include the above digestion-friendly meals and:

- A rotation of broth-based soups like fermented miso soup with seaweed and shiitake mushrooms, or with immune-building astragalus roots, increasingly adding more healthy foods as you get better. The warm broth will help loosen throat phlegm
- Boiled down, watery grain porridges, like juk (also called congee)
- Lightly steamed or blanched leafy greens, like cabbage, watercress, or spinach, with or without a small amount of dressing (homemade lemon and olive oil dressing), salt and pepper, or ghee and spices
- Easily digestible proteins, like roasted salmon with garlic
- Steamed or baked roots like radish, bamboo shoots, and leeks (you can also drink the cooking fluid) or sweet potato
- Warm fluids like warm water, or herbal teas with or without lemon to continue the cleaning-out process
- Warming elements like cinnamon, turmeric, scallions, garlic, and ginger, which have antiviral and antiseptic properties
- Celery juice, which reduces inflammation; it works most effectively on an empty stomach
- Natural therapies to help rid your body of toxins like adding a small amount of seaweed to your diet, or taking a hot Epsom salt bath
- Electrolytes, like coconut water or lemon-salt water (see page 104), to keep your body balanced and hydrated

Recovery recipes passed down in Asian culture

In Asian culture (as with other cultures that have retained their culinary traditions), it is common to use home remedies to treat various ailments that come with periods of trauma recovery, including post-childbirth, post-surgery, or, like me, for gut-repair periods. The importance placed on recovery from childbirth in Asian culture, for example, has been critical to helping both baby and mother to cement a strong parent-child bond but also to practice the critical skills needed for breastfeeding, which allows the baby to receive the most optimal form of nourishment in the early stages of life. Special foods for mothers, as listed below, help them replenish fluids and nutrients like calcium lost during birth and breastfeeding. Protein-rich foods are given to boost energy levels, help shrink the uterus, and heal the perineum. I was lucky to receive these nourishing foods and support from my family, who tirelessly made me gelatinous soups to stock up on so that I was able to breastfeed for a full year for both children. They also performed little miracles on other family members in their recovery periods, as when they fed loved ones with their special soups and astonished doctors with speedy recovery from surgery within a mere few days. These were recipes that were passed down in my family, including many soupy recipes that had benefits for collagen, blood circulation, detoxification, and bone health. In Asian culture, when a family member is sick, there is an inherent need to heal and love through nourishing food.

Green papaya and fish soup

In traditional Asian kitchens, there are always a vast range of nourishing soups filled with plant-diverse nutrients, collagen from the bones, protein from the meat, and digestive aids from the fruits. I was fed these soups copiously after I gave birth and used them to help various family members through their recovery periods post-hospital stays. This green papaya and fish soup, which is popular in Hong Kong, employs the fibers from the green papaya to nourish the body; the fibers bond to chemicals and other toxins, helping to flush them out of the body.

Recipe notes

Although the recipe only requires the fish head and bones, if you bought a whole fish and had the market fillet the flesh, you can add fish slices to the finished soup under gentle heat. Fish slices should be briefly marinated in a cornstarch slurry with a touch of soy sauce for flavor.

(recipe continues)

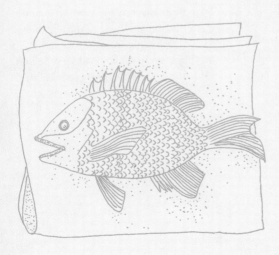

INGREDIENTS

Serves 8

1 pound fish head or fish bones from sea bass or red snapper

1 tablespoon toasted sesame oil

4 or 5 thin slices ginger

1 small green papaya (about 1 pound), peeled and cut into bite-sized pieces

4 dried jujubes

1 tablespoon goji seeds

4 garlic cloves, peeled (optional)

2 green onion stalks, cut into 2-inch segments (optional)

1½ teaspoons Hua Diao wine, similar to Shaoxine wine or sherry (optional)

Sea salt or pink Himalayan salt and freshly ground white pepper

METHOD

1. Clean the fish head and bones thoroughly with cold water and pat dry.

2. Heat the sesame oil in a large clay pot or stockpot over medium heat and add the ginger to infuse the oil. Add the fish heads and bones and cook lightly for 3 to 4 minutes per side. This is to remove the "fishiness" and keep the fish intact during cooking.

3. Add 5 cups of water, the papaya, jujubes, goji seeds, and, if using, the garlic, green onions, and wine.

4. Bring to a boil, then lower the heat and simmer for 1 hour. Remove from the heat and carefully strain the soup. Discard all the ingredients except the papaya. Return the papaya to the strained soup. Season with salt and white pepper before serving.

In my Korean household, we had our own household remedies (see page 193). Besides miyeokguk (seaweed soup) and kongnamul-guk (soybean sprout soup), a pared-down version of a monks' cold-remedy soup, my father would always make me samgyetang, a simple poached chicken soup, creating a stock with scallions, jujubes, garlic, and glutinous rice that would energize me. And when I was sick my mother would make me juk, a Korean staple for the sick, especially those with stomach ailments, made by slow-boiling rice, creating a soft texture that was easy to swallow and digest when I couldn't keep other foods down. My grandmother would make baesuk, poaching pears to make a tea with honey and ginger, which served as a remedy for a sore throat or cough. As a child, I took these dishes for granted, but I came to realize they were tangible representations of their love for me, and now this is what I do for my children, too.

Embarking on your reset

Before making any significant changes to your diet or overhauling your pantry, I would recommend that you first get a baseline assessment of your current health, using steps that you can take on your own and with the help of a trusted doctor. Diet and lifestyle choices affect each of us in very different ways, and there is no one-size-fits-all.

Gluten, dairy, soy, and grains are often touted as the common culprits of inflammation. However, these food items are not problematic for all of us, and in fact, they are eaten across many food cultures that support happy and healthy centenarians. The World Wildlife Fund, an outstanding nonprofit focused on conserving a healthy environment, does not believe in a "one-size-fits-all" diet. For them, healthy and sustainable diets should reflect the rich diversity of culinary traditions and needs around the world. Rather than following the latest diet trend and going gluten-free or dairy-free or Paleo, I encourage you to empower yourself. Learn more about your physiological makeup and make dietary choices that are ideal for your body and its unique needs.

Things you can do with a doctor:

- Consult an allergy specialist or functional doctor to take a food sensitivity test, which will tell you if you are sensitive to any foods and therefore should have less of them or not have them in your kitchen
- Have bloodwork done to check for any micronutrient deficiencies, like vitamin D, magnesium, or calcium, and check your cholesterol, blood sugar level, and cancer markers

Things you can do on your own:

- Listen to your body daily and keep a food journal (see page 206) to help find and track changes or reactions to certain foods
- Remove any food items that you know cause you inflammation or irritation from your pantry
- Stock your pantry and fridge with as many whole ingredients as possible
- Keep healthy foods visible and within easy access
- Consider batch cooking and freezing as ways to make your busy week healthy and easy

My Asian-inspired longevity pantry

FERMENTED FOODS

- [ ] **Doenjang** (Korean soybean paste)
- [ ] **Ganjang** (Korean soy sauce)
- [ ] **Gochujang** (Korean red chili paste)
- [ ] **Gukganjang** (Korean soup soy sauce)
- [ ] **Kimchi**
- [ ] **Miso** (Japanese soybean paste)
- [ ] **Natto** (Japanese soybeans)
- [ ] **Sauerkraut**
- [ ] **Ssamjang** (Korean gochujang and doenjang mixture)

VEGETABLES & FUNGI

- [ ] **Bitter melon, fresh and powdered**
- [ ] **Garlic, whole and pre-minced**
- [ ] **Ginger, fresh and powdered**
- [ ] **Ginseng, fresh and powdered**
- [ ] **Goguma** (Korean sweet potato)
- [ ] **Herbs** (e.g., coriander, parsley, cilantro, mint)
- [ ] **Kongnamul** (soybean sprouts)
- [ ] **Mu** (Korean radish)
- [ ] **Mushrooms** (e.g., shiitake)
- [ ] **Perilla** (Korean mint leaf)
- [ ] **Red leaf lettuce**
- [ ] **Scallion**
- [ ] **Seaweed** (e.g., kombu, miyeok, roasted sheets)
- [ ] **Shiso** (Japanese mint leaf)
- [ ] **Ssukgat** (garland chrysanthemum)
- [ ] **Seasonal vegetables**

FRUITS

- [ ] **Bae** (Korean pear)
- [ ] **Citrus** (e.g., lemon, lime, tangerines)
- [ ] **Gam** (persimmon), **fresh and dried**
- [ ] **Jujubes, dried**
- [ ] **Kabocha squash**
- [ ] **Monkfruit, dried**
- [ ] **Seasonal fruits**

SOUP BASES & SPICES

- [ ] **Anchovy soup bag with kombu, dried shrimp, anchovies, and shiitake**
- [ ] **Astragalus, powdered**
- [ ] **Bonito flakes**
- [ ] **Gochugaru** (Korean red chili flakes)
- [ ] **Meat or fish to make collagen broth or soups** (e.g., oxtail or yellow corvina fish)
- [ ] **Myeolchi** (dried anchovies)
- [ ] **Sea salt or pink Himalayan salt**
- [ ] **Other spices** (e.g., turmeric, cinnamon)

OTHER

- [ ] **Healthy oils** (e.g., sesame, coconut, olive oil)
- [ ] **Purple rice**
- [ ] **Ready-made banchan** (e.g., gosari, or brown bracken fern, doraji, or bellow flower root, or burdock root)
- [ ] **Seeds** (e.g., chia, flax, black and white sesame, pumpkin, sunflower)
- [ ] **Teas** (e.g., boricha, or roasted barley, Matcha)
- [ ] **Tofu**
- [ ] **Vinegars** (e.g., persimmon, rice, white, black, apple cider)
- [ ] **Natural condiments**

Korean Recovery Recipes

"A mother's cooking has the ability to heal both body and soul."

—*Unknown*

Baesuk (Korean pear with jujube), Korean cold remedy

Baesuk is a traditional Korean cold remedy with pears as its main ingredient. Pears are naturally hydrating—and water is a panacea for illnesses, especially when taken hot or warm. The pears are paired with vitamin-rich jujubes, cinnamon, ginger, and honey to make a delicious cold remedy that expels phlegm, eases sore throat and coughs, soothes the stomach, enhances metabolism, and cleanses the blood vessels.

Although you can use any variety of pear in this recipe, Korean pear (also known as Asian pear) is particularly beneficial. Compared to Bosc pears, Korean pears have lower sugar content, higher water content, and more dietary fiber, manganese, magnesium, and protein.[1] They are also quite delicious and my children's favorite fruit. I can hardly keep them in stock at home!

Recipe notes

Pears are good for the colon, containing chlorogenic acid, which is a bioactive ingredient also found in apples that helps boost metabolism and burn fat. It has also been shown to stop the growth of tumors. Baked pears are also recommended for lung and breathing ailments, as they can help with relieving phlegm and congestion.

Stewed pears, and apples as well, are particularly good for gut health. Eating them regularly can help with bloating and stomach issues. When pears are cooked, they release extra pectin, a form of fiber, which nourishes the gut bacteria.

Jujubes are packed with vitamins A, B_1, and B_2, and they contain twenty times the amount of vitamin C of citrus fruits. They also contain minerals that promote bone health, including magnesium, copper, manganese, and potassium.

INGREDIENTS

Serves 2

2 Korean pears (or any pear variety, like Bosc)

3 dried jujubes, chopped and seeded

½ teaspoon ground cinnamon

1 tablespoon grated fresh ginger

1 to 2 tablespoons honey, to taste (optional)

METHOD

1. Cut each pear at the top lengthwise, like a topper, keeping the skin on. Core to remove the seeds.

2. Fill 2 of the cored pear halves with the jujubes, cinnamon, ginger, and honey, if using. Place the 2 pear tops on top, creating 2 "whole" pears.

3. Place a steam rack or bowl in a medium pot with water, being careful that the water doesn't touch the rack. Carefully place the stuffed pears on the rack, set over low heat, cover, and steam for 1 hour, or until soft, making sure to check if you need to add more water to the pot.

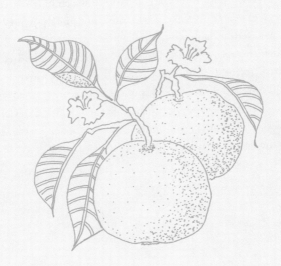

Juk (Korean porridge), a remedy for upset stomach

Whether for a loved one who has an upset stomach, has just returned home from the hospital, or is simply hungry, in a Korean household, the solution usually includes juk, also known as congee. A creamy, easily digestible dish of boiled rice, juk is typically served seasoned with sesame oil, soy sauce, sesame seeds, and scallion. It also provides a versatile base for a variety of dishes that include abalone, chicken, or pumpkin. Although it has ancient roots in Korean royal cuisine, juk is historically known for helping the average Korean household make rice stretch during financially challenging times.

Whenever I fell ill as a child, this was the remedy that my Korean mother prepared to help me get better, along with freshly washed bedsheets to lie in. Juk always calmed me and nourished my upset stomach when I couldn't keep anything down. I enjoyed juk so much growing up that it was the only dish I learned to make as a child. To this day, the nutty smell of sesame oil evokes my mother's love and the white Formica kitchen countertops in my childhood home.

Though this recipe serves two, it is easily scalable. Feel free to add to this basic recipe. I prefer to use already cooked or leftover rice to cut the recipe time and to add a cup of shredded chicken seasoned with garlic, sesame oil, salt, and pepper at the end. Or I'll cook finely chopped vegetables—carrot, celery, and mushrooms—to soften them, then add them to the rice after the liquid is visibly reduced.

INGREDIENTS

Serves 2
(easily scalable)

1 cup short-grain rice, cooked

3 cups chicken stock or
filtered water

½ cup chopped vegetables:
carrot, celery, mushrooms
(optional)

1½ teaspoons toasted
sesame oil

½ cup cooked chicken
(optional)

½ teaspoon gukganjang
(Korean soup soy sauce) or
other naturally brewed soy
sauce

1½ teaspoons sesame seeds,
for garnish (optional)

Scallion greens, chopped, for
garnish (optional)

METHOD

1. In a medium pot, bring the cooked
   rice and stock to boil over medium-
   high heat.

2. If using, add the carrots, celery, and
   mushrooms to the pot, bring to a
   simmer, then lower the heat and
   simmer, stirring, for another 10 to
   15 minutes, until the vegetables
   are softened and the stock is visibly
   reduced. Add the sesame oil to
   flavor the rice mixture.

3. If using cooked chicken, stir it
   in during the last few minutes of
   simmering.

4. Ladle into a bowl and top with the
   soy sauce and, if using, the sesame
   seeds and scallions.

Kongnamul-guk (soybean sprout soup), Korean hangover remedy

In Korea, kongnamul-guk is commonly believed to help with recovery from hangovers. Koreans love to drink when they socialize, but they also know that restorative foods bring back balance after excess drinking. Kongnamul, or soybean sprouts, contain two specific things that make it the perfect remedy for a quick recovery from too much drinking: arginine, which is known for its detoxifying effects on acetaldehyde, a toxic metabolite produced in alcohol metabolism in humans, and asparagusic acid,[2] which protects the liver. What's more, soybean sprouts, harvested just a few days after they germinate, are even more vitamin-rich than their mature plant selves.

Kongnamul have a crunchy texture and nutty taste, and they are a popular ingredient in many Korean dishes, including as a salad ingredient or simply prepared as a banchan. In Korea, kongnamul-guk is also considered a light and highly nutritious everyday soup to pair with your meals.

Recipe notes

Kongnamul are linked to numerous health benefits, like reducing the risk of cardiovascular diseases and cancer, from several health-promoting phytochemicals with high-antioxidant properties.[3] Kongnamul are also believed to assist digestion and promote a healthy gut microbiome while preventing and treating high blood pressure.

Kongnamul are rich in folate, vitamin K, protein, beta-carotene, lutein, vitamin C, vitamin B-complex, copper, and vitamin E.

INGREDIENTS

Serves 1
(easily scalable)

6 to 8 medium to large dried anchovies

1 plump garlic clove, thinly sliced

1 cup kongnamul (soybean sprouts)

Sea salt or pink Himalayan salt and freshly ground white pepper

1 scallion, green parts, chopped

METHOD

1. In a medium pot, combine 6 cups of filtered water, the anchovies, and garlic and bring to a boil over high heat. Reduce the heat to medium-high and continue to boil, uncovered, for 10 minutes. Fish out the anchovies and garlic from the broth (you can use a slotted spoon or ladle strainer) and discard.

2. Rinse the soybean sprouts, then add them to the pot along with 1 teaspoon salt. Lower the heat to medium, cover, and cook for an additional 5 minutes. Season with salt and pepper.

3. Garnish with the scallion and serve.

Doraji (bellflower root),
Korean cough relief

Doraji, also known as bellflower, balloon flower, or platycodon, grows wild in the mountains of Korea and blossoms into a beautiful, deep purple aster-shaped flower. It roots have long been used in herbal medicine in Korea as a home remedy for coughs and asthma, its bitter and fibrous qualities made edible by brewing them to make tea or softening them with water and sweetening them with honey or, for a more savory taste, toasted sesame oil or soy sauce.

According to *Dongui Bogam*, a medical book published in 1613 during the Joseon Dynasty, doraji is beneficial for increasing blood circulation in the lungs, thereby aiding with shortness of breath, sore throat, chest pain, and coughing. Doraji "is a medicine that acts like the oars of a boat by carrying all medicines and preventing them from going down and raising energy and blood."[4] Eating doraji can strengthen the lining of the bronchial tubes that become susceptible to infection during the polluted spring. The root also helps in expelling phlegm and soothing the lungs when they are overexposed to particulates. Research has also uncovered that doraji has bioactive compounds that exhibit antitumor, anti-inflammatory, and anti-diabetic activities.[5]

If you have ordered Korean bibimbap, a popular mixed vegetable rice bowl, it is likely that you have already tried doraji, which is a common ingredient in this dish, as well as in banchan. In Korea, you can easily find them pre-peeled and shredded in the markets or from street vendors. In the US, you can find the dried version in Korean markets or online. I didn't quite understand the value of doraji growing up, and now when I have the chance to get it, I really do savor this special root.

INGREDIENTS

Serves 1
(easily scalable)

2 ounces dried doraji

Honey

METHOD

1. In a bowl, soak the dried doraji in room temperature water to soften, about 1 hour. Drain and cut into matchsticks.

2. Add honey to taste to temper the bitterness.

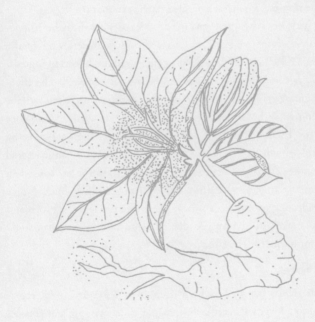

Samgyetang (chicken and ginseng soup), Korean antidote to fatigue

Samgyetang is a savory soup made with a whole small chicken stuffed with ginger, glutinous rice, garlic, and jujubes. In Korea, it is traditionally consumed on the three hottest days of the year. Although this may seem counterintuitive, Koreans believe the heat from the soup, along with the heating properties of ginger and ginseng, helps to regulate body temperature by producing sweat, which has a cooling effect. While popular in the summer, samgyetang is also eaten year-round.

Many cultures have their version of chicken soup, but the Korean version uniquely places significance on the medicinal powers of the ginseng broth, which combines with other immune-boosting ingredients like ginger and jujubes. Together, the soup is believed to be effective in increasing resistance to stress, helping to recover from fatigue, suppressing high blood pressure, and having an anti-inflammatory tonic effect. I adapted this soup to include another immune-boosting ingredient—dried astragalus root powder—which has antibacterial and anti-inflammatory properties. I made this soup for my son when he came out of surgery to help him recover. I also tend to make this dish at the beginning of the week so that I can use the leftover broth and chicken to make additional meals all week. It's a dish that my father used to make for me all the time, too.

Recipe notes

Glutinous rice is believed to help strengthen bone density, decrease inflammation, improve heart health, regulate diabetes, prevent chronic diseases, reduce inflammation, and optimize metabolism.

I keep dried ginger and dried astragalus root powders in my freezer at all times. They can last up to a year.

INGREDIENTS

Serves 4 to 6

1½ teaspoons ginseng, dried

1½ teaspoons astragalus, dried

2 scallions, white ends with roots for the soup, greens thinly sliced for garnish

1 whole young chicken (about 1½ pounds)

Sea salt or pink Himalayan salt

3 tablespoons sweet glutinous rice (if you have time, soak it in water for 30 minutes, then drain)

1-inch piece fresh ginger, with skin, sliced

4 garlic cloves (no need to peel)

6 dried jujubes

Freshly ground white pepper

METHOD

1. In a medium pot, combine 6½ cups of filtered water with the ginseng, astragalus, and the white part of the scallions with roots and bring to a boil over medium-high heat.

2. Wash the chicken including the cavity thoroughly with cold running water, then rub it with salt inside and out to help clean it. Do a final rinse of the chicken.

3. Stuff the chicken cavity with the sweet rice, ginger, garlic, and jujubes. Tie the legs together with butcher's twine to keep the ingredients from spilling out.

4. Add the stuffed chicken and enough filtered water to cover it in the pot, bring to a boil, then lower the heat a little, cover, and boil for 20 minutes. Reduce the heat to medium-low and simmer for about 30 minutes more, skimming off any scum, until the chicken is fully cooked.

5. Serve with salt, white pepper, and chopped scallions on the side, for each person to season and garnish to taste.

Listen to Your Body

"If you listen to your body when it whispers, you will never have to listen to it scream."

—Unknown

One of the key preventative health measures we can incorporate into our routines is to check in with our bodies daily—taking a quick scan from head to toe to check for any ailments or changes. If we notice something out of the ordinary, we can take the next step to reach out to the doctor, even if we have no obvious symptoms or current diagnosis. While doing this daily might seem extraneous, it only takes a few minutes and can help us to identify important changes that predate serious medical issues, like a malignant lump, or in my case, repeated abdominal pains, which I ignored and which led to my emergency room visit. Symptoms that show up in the body can be indicators of the overall state of our health.

When we experience injury to a part of the body, a signal travels through our nerves to the spinal cord where neurotransmitters are released, telling our brain that we are experiencing pain. When this pain is minor or temporary, we can often address it ourselves and the pain will go away. Minor headaches, for example, can often be remedied with a nap or more water intake. However, chronic headaches may be caused by inflammation or other problems with blood vessels in and around the brain, including stroke, infection, a brain tumor, or a traumatic brain injury.[1] In this case, you will want to listen to your body before your health worsens and consult your doctor right away.

Keep a food journal for a little while

A food journal is another tool for listening to your body. It is a log of what you eat and drink each day, along with any positive or negative

What your body might be telling you

	Healthy	Possible signs of an unhealthy state
Palms	Pinkish red with a shiny, smooth texture	Gray or lack of color
Hair	Growing and shiny	Lack of shine or luster (dull), hair loss
Skin	Feels comfortable without soreness, burning or itchiness; flesh-toned	Irregularly shaped or colored moles, gray or yellow skin, rashes, lumps
Nails	Smooth and pink	Brittle
Gastro-intestinal	Regular bowel movements daily	Nausea, vomiting, heartburn or reflux, constipation, bloating
Cardio fitness	Able to climb four flights of stairs without stopping;[2] healthy adults should have a resting heart rate of between 60 and 100 beats per minute	Chest pain, lightheadedness, fainting
Energy level	Energized	Chronically fatigued
Mental	Carrying a generally positive outlook	Chronic stress, depression, sadness, anxiety, feelings of helplessness

symptoms that might occur. This is a simple and effective tool to use for one to two weeks when you are just starting out with a mind to improve your health. Prior to my health journey, I had not heard about food journals.

A food journal can help you be more aware of how you consume and point to helpful information from your eating habits; for example, stomach pains that occur after having dairy products. It's like backtracking your steps to find your lost keys. Once you identify patterns, you can change your diet to improve your health and well-being.

When I kept a food journal, I noticed that on the days I didn't allow my body enough time to digest my dinners before breakfast, I experienced interrupted sleep that broke the eight hours my body tends to need to feel energized when I wake up. Now I know that an ideal day for me would be to allow two to three hours of post-dinner digestion, with no food, just water or herbal tea, and an evening stroll before sleep.

The origins of the food journal in Korea

In Korea, one might say that the origins of the food journal date back to the Joseon Dynasty, when the king requested a trusted royal physician to organize the existing medicinal knowledge that originated from China. He compiled all known medical texts, traditional remedies, and herbal medicine passed down through generations into a twenty-five-volume medical encyclopedia known as the *Dongui Bogam*, which literally means "priceless book about medicines of an Eastern Country." At the time, this ancient encyclopedia was the most complete body of work for the traditional use of functional foods and remedies in Korea. Its volumes classified fruits, vegetables, seafood, minerals, jades, metals, insects, plants, herbs, mushrooms, grains, and other naturally available raw materials with practical applications to remedy affected body parts. The existence of the *Dongui Bogam* confirms the generally accepted view in Asia that food was treated as medicine and was recorded for its positive and adverse reactions to the body, forming the basis for the food journals later kept by palace physicians for the ancient kings.

Commonly known ingredients like walnuts, apples, and spinach are listed alongside exotic ingredients like mugwort and chickweed. And though this dossier is ancient, surprisingly, much of the knowledge is still valuable and relevant in modern times. For example, the hawthorn berry fruit, with its leaves and flowers, is recorded in the *Dongui Bogam* as a plant that "resolves food accumulation and . . . removes blood stasis that has turned into mass, phlegmy spit and accumulation . . . wash it with water and steam it until it is soft . . . after that, remove the seed and dry it under the sun";[3] this still holds true, as contemporary studies show the apple-tasting hawthorn to help relieve digestive, heart, and blood pressure problems. Many studies have linked hawthorn with antioxidant, anti-inflammatory, anticancer, anticardiovascular disease, and digestive-enhancing properties.

Today, the *Dongui Bogam* is included in UNESCO's Memory of the World Program, and the original edition is preserved in the Korean National Library as an ancient manuscript demonstrating the historic importance of functional foods in Korea.

Jeong:
The
Invisible
Embrace

In Korean culture, each child is protected by an
expanding quilt of heartwarming experiences shared
with the people, places, or things that touch their life,
much like an invisible embrace. In Korean culture,
this is called jeong.

My father gifted me an old photo of himself as a reminder of what he looked like in his youth. In his furrowed eyebrows, full lips, and square jaw, I see my own face looking back. This is what my father's friends and family see, too, whenever I visit them in Korea. This face, which I inherited from my father, always prompts them to share fond memories of him. It reminds them of the invisible embrace, the jeong, that wrapped them together with my father over the years. This jeong still connects them, transcending time and space, now that my father lives and works as a doctor in New York, where he may spend his remaining years.

During my last trip to Seoul, my father's best friend, Dr. Choi, tirelessly escorted me throughout the city. He and my father graduated from Seoul National University College of Medicine together, and they both love to reminisce about their school days as ambitious young lads ready to take on the world. Because of the jeong that Dr. Choi has with my father, he offers to take care of my entire trip to Korea and meticulously plans out every minute detail for my research while I am there. He worries about my safety and my ability to travel independently, and he asks me to text him when I return to my hotel at the end of each day. Perhaps my uncanny resemblance and my connection to my father reminds Dr. Choi of the jeong they share, encouraging him to extend the kindness and warm feelings that he has for my father to me. I am the reincarnation of the dear friend he has not seen for decades.

For Koreans, jeong dul da means "jeong permeates," and it seeps into the smallest of daily interactions. If you ever watch a Korean film or TV show, pay attention and you will notice the innocent, playful quality of jeong. Jeong exists in giving the best pieces of your meal to a loved one. It is sharing a Choco Pie, the popular chocolate marshmallow cookie sandwich. It is friends singing noraebang karaoke all night over shots of soju. It is a stranger giving up their seat on the train or lending a handkerchief to someone in need. It is giving without expecting anything in return. Each of these acts of kindness builds jeong. Once it is formed, jeong will always exist somewhere in the depths of one's psyche, no matter how long it's been since one has seen the person, place, or thing since bonding through jeong, like an indelible permanent marker that can never be erased.

We might think of jeong as a nourishing soup with the most inexplicably complex flavors. The word evokes a distinctly Korean range of emotions—there is no equivalent in English. Jeong goes deeper and is far more complex than a simple hug or kiss, or even love at first sight. **Jeong is many things at once—love, friendship, empathy, compassion, sincerity, loyalty, sacrifice, community, connection, vulnerability, affection, sympathy, warmth, passion, kindness, social responsibility, and generosity of spirit toward humankind.** As a Korean American, understanding jeong allowed me to better understand my older, more traditional family members whose emotions run deep but who do not express their feelings toward me in the usual Western ways, through hugs or words. I have come to grasp how deeply they care for me in their way, an altered perspective that has caused me to think twice about different meanings across cultures.

Toward the end of my trip to Korea, Dr. Choi introduced me to Dr. Park, a well-known longevity expert who was also a classmate and has spent much of his career studying longevity patterns in Korea. I asked Dr. Park if he thought jeong was part of Korea's collective good health and well-being.

"My dear, jeong is the most important part of it all."

The psychology of jeong

In Korea, public displays of affection are uncommon; instead, there is jeong, which goes beyond the physical. Jeong is so ingrained in Korean culture that there is an entire set of vocabulary derived from it: mojeong is the love and affection of a mother; bujeong is love and affection of a father; aejeong is romantic love between two people; woojeong is friendship; miunjeong is the affectionate mixture of hatred and love that occurs in rivalry. The very idea of such an expansive concept serves as a collective call to Koreans, even if they are strangers, to help one another in the deepest way possible through shared trials and victories. Jeong gives us the language and the goal for creating the deep emotional bonds we all strive for to stay connected as human beings.

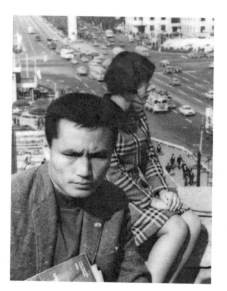

MY FATHER CAPTURED BY THE *CHOSUN ILBO*, A MAJOR NEWSPAPER IN KOREA, DURING HIS STUDENT COUNCIL PRESIDENCY FOR SEOUL NATIONAL UNIVERSITY COLLEGE OF MEDICINE

In Korea, there tends to be a rapid collective response to band together when there is a hardship or societal need. This is jeong in action and is evident throughout Korea's history. In the wake of the 1997 Asian financial crisis, South Koreans gathered gold jewelry from their own homes and donated over two billion dollars worth to help pay down the national IMF debt. In 2013, in response to what they saw as a national waste crisis, the South Korean government implemented mandates to recycle and compost leftover food. Citizens quickly responded, effectively wiping out food waste in the country. Jeong was also integral in Korea's response to containing the COVID-19 outbreak, with citizens demonstrating unified cooperation in contact tracing, masking, and isolation. Every member of Korean society, even children and the elderly, is seen as an integral part of the social fabric and therefore responsible for helping others if they can. In the words of journalist Daniel Tudor, "Jeong creates a kind of unwritten contract, the promise of help whenever it is needed."

When I was growing up, I cherished a children's book that told an old Korean folktale, "Heungbu and Nolbu." I was enchanted by its unique illustrations, and the bright yellow cover became frayed from reading the book many times. Now, I understand that I was learning ideas of jeong that my parents were trying to instill in me. In the tale, Heungbu, the kinder of two brothers, comes upon a baby swallow with a broken leg. Heungbu protects the swallow from a snake, and brings the swallow back home to care for it until it is strong enough to fly. After three days, the swallow returns with a gift—a seed—which grows into three remarkably large pumpkins. When Heungbu cuts the pumpkins open, he is shocked to find within them riches and treasures beyond his imagination. The swallow has rewarded Heungbu for his generosity, kindness of spirit, and good-naturedness, jeong traits and values that are revered and taught in Korean culture.

The idea of jeong continues to be reinforced and passed down through folktales like these, family conversations, and popular culture. If you watch a commercial in Korea or K-drama, you'll notice jeong traits in the most loved characters portrayed. It is apt that swallows represent love, loyalty, help, and new beginnings. This is what jeong is—a chance to start anew, even with the people who are already in your life, with kindheartedness and a warm gesture.

Jeong-based values are related to other Korean concepts; for example, woori and nunchi. Woori (us/our) is used as a preceding term for other words in the Korean language. Koreans refer to their country as woori nara (our country), or immediate family members as entities who are shared with others, as in woori umma (our mother) or woori ahbuhji (our father); they are means to establish an immediate rapport and connection with others. Nunchi is the concept of developing an exceptional sense of emotional intelligence, the ability to gauge a sensitivity to others' moods in order to create harmony in interpersonal relationships. These concepts show how Korean culture is postured toward a connected society.

When viewing Korean society, UCLA Medical Center psychiatrists Dr. Cho and Dr. Chung, graduates of Seoul National University College of Medicine and UC Davis School of Medicine, suggest that in Korean culture, there is a reorder of Maslow's hierarchy of needs, a well-known psychological framework that places basic physiological needs, including food, shelter, and clothing, first as a foundation. Dr. Cho and Dr. Chung believe that jeong comes first in Korean society because of its emphasis on belonging and community.[1] Jeong encourages everyone to view each other as part of one big family, each member caring for one another. No one gets left behind.

Relationships are the greatest health predictors

In 1938, researchers at Harvard University began tracking the health of 268 Harvard sophomores in an ongoing, groundbreaking study that is one of the world's longest health studies of adult life. Robert Waldinger, professor of psychiatry at Harvard Medical School and the current director of the study, expanded the research to include the children of the original research subjects, and published a book, *The Good Life*,[2] on the findings. Research participants were analyzed through extensive medical records, in-person interviews, and questionnaires, along with detailed measures of brain activity, DNA testing, and MRI scans, along with the successes and failures of their marriages, career trajectories, and even their handwriting.

When the study began, researchers postulated that happiness and contentment in life would largely be determined by physical constitution, intellectual ability, and personality traits. However, as the study progressed, findings revealed that the quality and presence of close relationships in a person's life are better predictors of longevity, happiness, and health than measures like cholesterol, IQ, social class, or fame. According to Waldinger, "Taking care of your body is important, but tending to your relationships is a form of self-care too." These ties are believed "to protect people from life's discontents, and help delay mental and physical decline."[3] For Waldinger, "The good life is built with good relationships."

Similarly, with its focus on building deep, community-level connection, jeong binds Koreans together to build on strong relationships. Jeong would seem to be the antidote to social isolation and loneliness, factors that rival smoking, obesity, alcoholism, and physical inactivity in increasing a person's risk for dementia and premature death.[4]

Jeong as a code to live by

One day in Seoul, I had a chance to reconnect for a meal with relatives who I hadn't seen for many years, since I was a teenager. I really enjoyed meeting cousins who were no longer babies and seeing what they had become. Gunwan, for example, who had always been considered ttogttog (smart), was now an engineer at Samsung. When I saw my aunt Misook-Komo, a doppelganger to my father and me, she rushed to me. "Aigu, Michelle-y-yah!" She squeezed my arm tightly as if no time had passed, while we downloaded on happenings in our family. I mentioned how much I liked her beads, and she immediately took them off her neck and put them on mine. Still warm to the touch, they felt like a tangible piece of the jeong that would always be there between us. I instantly felt so much love.

I think about my relatives in Korea whenever I go to K-town in Midtown Manhattan and H Mart to stock up on Korean ingredients. On my visits there, I feel jeong with the community that H Mart brings— for those Koreans who have immigrated to a foreign place, for those who enjoy Korean food, and for people like me who are trying to learn more about Korean culture. Grocers like H Mart replicate the basement floor of department stores that I used to visit with my parents in Korea, filled with ahjummas (older women) donning aprons and rubber gloves, spooning heaps of banchan for you. The recollections all intermingle into the jeong I feel for my Korean family.

Whenever I go to H Mart, I read the Korean words on all the labels, searching for more meaning to the homeland of my family, searching for the connection to my cultural identity that I had gradually let go of. I find community in people who similarly understand my requirements for large packages of dried seaweed and vats of minced garlic. Only in Korean grocers like H Mart will I find wellness products like heating pads, UV sun visors, boricha (roasted barley tea), and samgyetang (ginseng root–chicken soup) kits without thinking of their foreign placements next to each other.

One day, on my way to K-town, I helped a man who fell, the items from his shopping bag spilling out onto the floor. I thought about how this was standard behavior for people who use jeong as a code to live by, and I tried to embody jeong more often. I doubled down on my work with mission-driven organizations. I made a point of holding doors, offering smiles, and chatting with strangers. I reconnected with long-lost friends on social media. I tried to have deeper conversations with loved ones. I realized that I had been forgetting to make the time for these kind gestures during my busy day-to-day.

I also worked to improve jeong within—being kinder and gentler with myself, especially when things go wrong. These days, appreciating the little things that I am able to achieve and, of course, self-care in all its forms are vital aspects of my day. My jeong practice is still a work in progress, but I find that it makes me feel happier and more connected with others at the end of each day.

I will always have lifelong jeong with certain people who have been important in my life, like my Harvard Business School fellows, especially my Section D classmates, who collectively WhatsApp me all the time. Or friends from childhood who knew me back when I had braces and curly hair. The haenyeo will always have jeong with each other. And my Buddhist friend, Minh, will always have jeong in the social fabric of his religious community, which for him extends to the global network of temples to his Korean Buddhist practice.

For Koreans, jeong is not meant to be defined so much as experienced. It awakens a sense of familiarity and comfort, and at its core, jeong is about magnanimous giving without expecting anything in return. Some say that it is equivalent to altruism. Here are a few examples of how jeong might manifest, even in what might seem the smallest possible ways:

- Sharing a snack with another
- Helping someone to carry a heavy bag
- Giving up your seat on the bus or subway
- Bringing food to welcome someone new in your community
- Offering an unsolicited smile to a stranger to spread kindness
- Having concern over others' well-being; ensuring even acquaintances are dressed warmly or have had enough water or food that day, for example

Jeong is a free and easy attitude that we can all adopt to boost our well-being. While the extent of this word is uniquely Korean, the idea is one that is practiced in different degrees across the world and that we can all tap into. Although the essence of jeong is to send good energy into the world without expecting rewards in return, studies do show that empathy, kindness, compassion, and service—all elements of jeong— have significant physiological and psychological benefits, including decreasing blood pressure and levels of the stress hormone cortisol in the body. Jeong is like a gift basket of wide-ranging warm feelings, like an invisible embrace, and it has the ability to trigger multiple "happy" hormones, including serotonin, which promotes feelings of calm and happiness; dopamine, which promotes pleasure and reward; and oxytocin, which promotes love and affection. And if we form jeong while laughing, exercising, or spending time outdoors, we are also producing endorphins, the fourth "happy" hormone, known as the body's natural painkiller. When we use jeong as a code for living, as the Koreans do, we build robust relationships, feel a deeper sense of belonging, and find healthy outlets for our bodies and brains to respond to challenging situations that invariably come with living a full life.

Passing Traditions On

On my dol, my first birthday, I was bedecked in a hanbok (a traditional Korean outfit) and a golden crown with dangling beads that framed my chubby cheeks. Much like the baek-il celebrating the hundredth day, the dol is steeped in Korean tradition, for it represents an important milestone that signifies a baby's survival. It is customary to have stacks of colorful food, rainbow-layered tteok (rice cakes), and bowls filled decadently with all sorts of beautiful fruit. It is a feast for the eyes and belly, an abundant display of food meant to give blessings that the baby will never go hungry. And the main activity for this first birthday is doljabi, a game in which the celebrated baby chooses from a range of items to "predict" its potential calling in life.

In accordance with this old tradition, I was placed in front of a series of objects with special significance to our family to choose from; my choice would signify how my life might eventually unfold. If I grabbed my father's golf ball in front of me, I might become a golfer or an athlete. If I chose a stethoscope, I would be a doctor like him. If I favored the pencil, I would be an educator like my grandfather. According to my parents, I hovered over the bowl of rice grains and the dollar bill. Eventually, I chose the rice. How funny and appropriate that I decided on the very thing that symbolized a long and prosperous life and that I have now written a book on the very subject.

Throughout my childhood, there were glimmers of Korean traditions like my dol that were special and memorable. But as I grew up, I increasingly wanted to blend in with the Western culture I was being raised in and I began to adopt more of the conveniences and features of modern life. Whenever my family took trips to visit American landmarks like Disneyland, I couldn't contain my excitement. I liked to eat hot dogs and breakfast cereals with food coloring and drink boxed orange juice. After a while, I had forgotten to practice the Korean traditions I grew up with. The language of my native culture and the wild greens and seaweeds, things that were normalized in my early childhood, all faded into the background.

Every culture has its own set of traditional wisdom that can be preserved, honored, and even adapted to what makes sense in their generation. Today, as my children grow up living between cultures in Asia and the US, I am mindful of passing along generational knowledge and what I have learned through my health journey. I want them to inherit

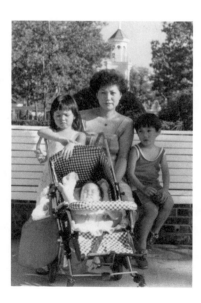

WITH MOM AT
DISNEYLAND
LIVING THE
QUINTESSENTIAL
AMERICAN EXPERIENCE

and benefit from the wisdom of their native cultures, which for them are both Korean and Chinese, and healthfully make them their own.

One of my greatest achievements on this journey was being able to change the mind of my son, who was at one time most obstinate in his eating habits. I knew something big was happening when one day my son sat down at the table with a meal that he had made for himself—a bowl filled with mushroom soup and purple rice from our refrigerator, a side of cilantro topping and raw perilla leaves left over from the night before, with a final squeeze of half a lemon on top. He hadn't thought twice about throwing these ingredients together. I realized that he was grasping the benefits of eating a plant-diverse diet after months of listening to me talk about my trips and my learnings.

Then, on another morning, I woke to the clanging of pots down the hall and found that my son and daughter were working together in the kitchen to prepare a simple, healthy breakfast: a vegetable-filled omelet with a side of fruit and sesame sprinkled namul. They were helping each other to plate and cook, using whatever was in the refrigerator to make a meal, not wanting to waste it. They sat down to eat and talk with each other in an unexpected and delightfully heartwarming scene of what I now know in Korean culture as jeong, the invisible tie that will bind them forever together.

I stared at them in wonder, knowing that a beautiful transformation had occurred in our family. Before my hospitalization, I would never have been able to prepare these types of meals, but it was evident that my children had learned along with me as I discovered time-honored remedies to heal naturally. I hope this helps to set them on a path to leading healthier lives while reconnecting with the ancient wisdom of our ancestors. I hope, too, that they pass these traditions on to their children.

These days, I know it's necessary for me to take breaks from the business of life. I walk outdoors and smile more. I like to carry vinegars, soups, or fruit wherever I go. I pickle, and I ferment, too. I know it's all the little things that add up to the big things. I do things to respect my self-care. I discovered that I have the gift of time if I take care of my mind, body, and spirit.

Our latest home project is a tabletop planter, a narrow rectangle just big enough to accommodate a rotation of herbs and perilla leaves grown with seeds from Lani's Farm. Now that we have our little garden, it's easy to see the time, energy, and care that goes into growing this food. It's a massive departure from the days when my diet consisted mainly of takeout. I still eat out and enjoy the dining scene, but I like to eat in together with my family more.

And together we are choosing to eat the whole plant, which means so many things to us as a family now.

Acknowledgments

To bring a book to light, it takes a certain lived history with its ups and downs and the people who have touched your life, for they bring with them the joys, the lessons, and the inspiration. My deepest gratitude goes to:

My parents, for bringing me life, and for patiently answering my endless questions about our Korean origins.

Richard, for his encouragement and patience through my insatiable curiosity about everything and anything. Thank you for being my life partner, for your thoughtful counsel, and for the beautiful broths and plates of food that kept magically appearing at my desk while I wrote and drew for hours and healed.

Elliot and Amber, for enthusiastically experimenting and learning with me, testing every recipe, and trying all the new things with Mama. You gave me hope and confidence in my book ideas and that together we could preserve and carry forward what is good in our cultural traditions to the next generation.

Holly Faulks at Greene & Heaton, who was the first agent to believe in me and helped me send my book on a whirlwind adventure, resulting in an unbelievable outcome for this first-time author—with auctions and simultaneous deals across the world. Also, many thanks to her team, Kate Rizzo, Imogen Morrell, and Mia Dakin.

Lucinda Halpern at Lucinda Literary, who deftly took me through an incredibly exciting bidding auction in the US, together with Jackie Ashton.

Bernadette Marron at Piatkus, for being the first editor to sign on, and for her editorial vision, which encouraged me to express myself fully not only through my words but also through my illustrations and Korean heritage.

Sarah Kwak at Harvest, for being my fellow Korean American who innately understood the journey I went through reconnecting with my cultural identity and for her skillful edits. Also, many thanks to Melissa Lotfy, who pulled together all the design pieces beautifully to bring this home, and to Jacqueline Quirk, Amanda Hong, and Leda Scheintaub. And to Marta Schooler and Lynne Yeamans, who first took this on at HarperDesign.

Tanja Rauch at DuMont Buchverlag, Sofia Marchand at Planeta, and Raffaello Avanzini at Newton Compton, for enthusiastically signing on for book translations, in German, Spanish, and Italian, to share this book in their parts of the world, even prior to publication.

Jessica Sindler, for keeping me on track, testing book concepts with me, and helping my ideas to shine.

Susan Montgomery, Kara Adamson, Pete McIntosh, Simon Shaw, and the rest of the team at Hampton Agency, for believing in the book vision and bringing sophisticated creativity to this book, in which the design and illustrations eventually became as important as the words.

My beta readers, who read the entirety of my book at various points of development: Tracey Thomm, Soo Jung Hyun, Chef Naila Varawalla, and my brilliant sister and confidante, Dr. Erica Bang.

Those who helped push this book along at critical junctures: various faculty and alums of the Seoul National University College of Medicine, including my father, Dr. Joon J. Bang, Dr. Sang Chul Park, MD, PhD, and Dr. Yong Choi; Ven. Jeong Kwan Seunim, the Hwang Family at Ojina; Chef Hooni Kim of Meju and Little Banchan Shop; Suzy Kim; Steve and Eugena Kwang at Lani's Farm; Su and James Chen; Lucia Cho and the Gaon family; Dr. Sears Wellness Institute; the Academy of Healing Nutrition; Ming Chen; Janice Y.K. Lee; Alison Jahncke;

Dania Shawwa; Jean Kim; Ken Watanabe; Therese Tee and her grandmother Mrs. Cheng Li Shuk Kam ("Mama"); Dr. Minh Tran; Susan Shapiro; Peter Guzzardi; Lisa Tener; Ambre Morvan; my research survey responders; and countless others whom I met on my journey and shared valuable insights, each paving a new path.

My fellows in social impact at GrowNYC, BMABHK, The Chivas Venture, HKIS, ATEC, and my formidable Hong Kong book club, for continuing to inspire me to be a part of a more sustainable, wholesome, and equitable world.

And last but not least, my Korean and Chinese families, for always showing me the warmth and wisdom of our Asian heritage. It is only now that I understand and see what you were doing.

Notes

Introduction

1. United Nations Population Division, "Life Expectancy at Birth, Total (Years)," World Bank Open Data, 2022. https://data.worldbank.org/indicator/SP.DYN.LE00.IN.
2. Vasilis Kontis, et al., "Future Life Expectancy in 35 Industrialised Countries: Projections with a Bayesian Model Ensemble," *Lancet* 389, no. 10076 (February 21, 2017): 1323–35. https://doi.org/10.1016/s0140-6736(16)32381-9.

Buddhist Nuns & the Microbiome

1. Garnett Cheney, "Vitamin U Therapy of Peptic Ulcer," *California Medicine* (October 1952). https://www.ncbi.nlm.nih.gov/pmc/articles/PMC1521464/.
2. David R. Montgomery and Anne Biklé, *The Hidden Half of Nature: The Microbial Roots of Life and Health* (W. W. Norton & Company, 2016).
3. Lawrence A. David et al., "Diet Rapidly and Reproducibly Alters the Human Gut Microbiome," *Nature* 505, no. 7484 (2013): 559–63. https://doi.org/10.1038/nature12820.
4. M. Vizzotto et al., "Polyphenols of Selected Peach and Plum Genotypes Reduce Cell Viability and Inhibit Proliferation of Breast Cancer Cells While Not Affecting Normal Cells," *Food Chemistry* 164 (2014a), 363–70. https://doi.org/10.1016/j.foodchem.2014.05.060.

The Whole Plant: A Zero-Waste Approach

1. Slatnar Ana et al., "Response of the Phenylpropanoid Pathway to *Venturia inaequalis* Infection in Maturing Fruit of 'Braeburn' Apple," *Journal of Horticultural Science and Biotechnology* 85, no. 6 (November 7, 2015): 465–72. https://doi.org/10.1080/14620316.2010.11512699.
2. Data retrieved for 100g raw apple with skin. U.S. Department of Agriculture (April 1, 2019), FoodData Central Search Results. https://fdc.nal.usda.gov/fdc-app.html#/food-details/171688/nutrients; Data retrieved for 100g raw apple without skin. U.S. Department of Agriculture (April 1, 2019), FoodData Central Search Results. https://fdc.nal.usda.gov/fdc-app.html#/food-details/171689/nutrients.

3. Data retrieved for 100g boiled potato with skin. U.S. Department of Agriculture (April 1, 2019), FoodData Central Search Results. https://fdc.nal.usda.gov/fdc-app.html#/food-details/170438/nutrients; Data retrieved for 100g boiled potato without skin. U.S. Department of Agriculture (April 1, 2019), FoodData Central Search Results. https://fdc.nal.usda.gov/fdc-app.html#/food-details/170440/nutrients.

4. Heather Norman-Burgdolf, "Fruit and Vegetable Peels Contain Many Nutrients," *Exclusives*, Martin-Gatton College of Agriculture (September 30, 2021). https://exclusives.ca.uky.edu/2021/fcs/fruit-and-vegetable-peels-contain-many-nutrients.

5. Judith A. Marlett and Tsui-Fun Cheung, "Database and Quick Methods of Assessing Typical Dietary Fiber Intakes Using Data for 228 Commonly Consumed Foods," *Journal of the Academy of Nutrition and Dietetics* 97, no. 10 (1997): 1139–51. https://doi.org/10.1016/s0002-8223(97)00275-7; Shahnaz Alvi et al., "Effect of Peeling and Cooking on Nutrients in Vegetables," *Pakistan Journal of Nutrition* 2, no. 3 (2003): 189–91. https://doi.org/10.3923/pjn.2003.189.191; Changjiang Guo et al., "Antioxidant Activities of Peel, Pulp and Seed Fractions of Common Fruits as Determined by FRAP Assay," *Nutrition Research* 23, no. 12 (December 12, 2003): 1719–26. https://doi.org/10.1016/j.nutres.2003.08.005.

6. Hanna Leontowicz et al., "Comparative Content of Some Bioactive Compounds in Apples, Peaches and Pears and Their Influence on Lipids and Antioxidant Capacity in Rats," *Journal of Nutritional Biochemistry* 13, no. 10 (2002): 603–10. https://doi.org/10.1016/s0955-2863(02)00206-1.

Royal Cuisine & Plant Diversity

1. Daniel McDonald, Embriette Hyde, Justine W. Debelius, James T. Morton, Antonio Gonzalez, Gail Ackermann, Alexander A. Aksenov, et al. "American Gut: An Open Platform for Citizen Science Microbiome Research," *MSystems* 3, no. 3 (June 26, 2018). https://doi.org/10.1128/msystems.00031-18.

2. Data retrieved for 100g perilla. "Calories in Perilla," Calorie Slism (n.d.). https://slism.com/calorie/106095/#foodDataDetail; Data retrieved for 100g broccoli. "Calories in Broccoli," Calorie Slism (n.d.). https://slism.com/calorie/106263/#foodDataDetail.

3. Data retrieved for 100g raw persimmon. U.S. Department of Agriculture (April 1, 2019), FoodData Central Search Results. https://fdc.nal.usda.gov/fdc-app.html#/food-details/169941/nutrients; Data retrieved for 100g raw apple. U.S. Department of Agriculture (April 1, 2019), FoodData

Central Search Results. https://fdc.nal.usda.gov/fdc-app.html#/food-details/171689/nutrients.

Sunshine, Fresh Air & Dirt

1. Wayne Fields, *What the River Knows: An Angler in Midstream* (University of Chicago Press, 1996).
2. Else S. Bosman et al., "Skin Exposure to Narrow Band Ultraviolet (UVB) Light Modulates the Human Intestinal Microbiome," *Frontiers in Microbiology* 10 (October 23, 2019). https://doi.org/10.3389/fmicb.2019.02410.
3. Robynne Chutkan, *The Microbiome Solution* (Avery, 2016).

Daily Habits for Longevity

1. Kim Yon-se, "More than 10,000 Centenarians Reside in Seoul Metropolitan Area," *Korea Herald* (August 5, 2019). https://www.koreaherald.com/view.php?ud=20190805000182#:~:text=Seoul%20had%20the%20largest%20population,South%20Jeolla%20Province%20(794).
2. A. Prüss-Ustün et al., "Preventing Disease through Healthy Environments," World Health Organization (September 13, 2018). https://apps.who.int/iris/bitstream/handle/10665/204585/9789241565196_eng.pdf?sequence=1.
3. Yoonkyung Chang et al., "Improved Oral Hygiene Care Is Associated with Decreased Risk of Occurrence for Atrial Fibrillation and Heart Failure: A Nationwide Population-based Cohort Study," *European Journal of Preventive Cardiology* 27, no. 17 (November 2020), 1835–45. https://doi.org/10.1177/2047487319886018.

Longevity Meals

1. Alpana P. Shukla et al., "Food Order Has a Significant Impact on Postprandial Glucose and Insulin Levels," American Diabetes Association, *Diabetes Care* 38, no. 7 (July 1, 2015). https://doi.org/10.2337/dc15-0429.

The Life-Changing Benefits of Walking

1. Tim Althoff et al., "Large-Scale Physical Activity Data Reveal Worldwide Activity Inequality," *Nature* 547, no. 7663 (2017): 336–39. https://doi.org/10.1038/nature23018.
2. Aidan J. Buffey et al., "The Acute Effects of Interrupting Prolonged Sitting Time in Adults with Standing and Light-Intensity Walking on Biomarkers of Cardiometabolic Health in Adults: A Systematic Review and Meta-

Analysis," *Sports Medicine*, SpringerLink 52 (February 11, 2022). https://link.springer.com/article/10.1007/s40279-022-01649-4.

3. Junyeon Won, Kristy A. Nielson, and J. Carson Smith, "Large-Scale Network Connectivity and Cognitive Function Changes after Exercise Training in Older Adults with Intact Cognition and Mild Cognitive Impairment," *Journal of Alzheimer's Disease Reports* 7, no. 1 (May 12, 2023): 399–413. https://doi.org/10.3233/adr-220062.

4. Ciao-Lin Ho, Wei-Fong Wu, and Yiing Mei Liou, "Dose–Response Relationship of Outdoor Exposure and Myopia Indicators: A Systematic Review and Meta-Analysis of Various Research Methods," *International Journal of Environmental Research and Public Health* 16, no. 14 (July 21, 2019): 2595. https://doi.org/10.3390/ijerph16142595.

Haenyeo: Stewards of the Sea

1. American Lung Association, "Breathing Exercises," accessed November 17, 2022. https://www.lung.org/lung-health-diseases/wellness/breathing-exercises.

Hydration Culture

1. Thich Nhat Hanh, *The Miracle of Mindfulness: An Introduction to the Practice of Meditation* (Beacon Press, 1999). Copyright © 1975, 1976 by Thich Nhat Hanh.Preface and English translation Copyright © 1975, 1976, 1987 by Mobi Ho. Reprinted with permission from Beacon Press, Boston Massachusetts.

2. Mengshi Yi et al., "Tea Consumption and Health Outcomes: Umbrella Review of Meta-Analyses of Observational Studies in Humans," *Molecular Nutrition & Food Research* 63, no. 16 (July 2, 2019). https://doi.org/10.1002/mnfr.201900389.

3. Yi et al., "Tea Consumption and Health Outcomes"; Dana Loomis et al., "Carcinogenicity of Drinking Coffee, Mate, and Very Hot Beverages," *Lancet Oncology* 17, no. 7 (June 15, 2016): 877–78. https://doi.org/10.1016/s1470-2045(16)30239-x.

Jjimjilbang: Traditional Bathhouses

1. Nikolai A. Shevchuk, "Adapted Cold Shower as a Potential Treatment for Depression," *Medical Hypotheses* 70, no. 5 (2008): 995–1001. https://doi.org/10.1016/j.mehy.2007.04.052.

2. Joy Hussain and Marc Cohen, "Clinical Effects of Regular Dry Sauna

Bathing: A Systematic Review," *Evidence-Based Complementary and Alternative Medicine* 2018 (April 24, 2018): 1–30. https://doi.org /10.1155/2018/1857413.

3. "America's #1 Health Problem," American Institute of Stress, January 4, 2017. https://www.stress.org/americas-1-health-problem#:~:text=It%20 has%20been%20estimated%20that,are%20for%20stress%20related%20 problems.

4. Haemin Sunim, *The Things You Can See Only When You Slow Down: How to Be Calm in a Busy World* (Penguin, 2017).

My Holistic Approach to Healing

1. David Servan-Schreiber, *Anticancer: A New Way of Life* (Scribe Publications, 2010).

2. Gabor Maté, *When the Body Says No: The Cost of Hidden Stress* (Vermilion, 2019).

3. Bessel van der Kolk, *The Body Keeps the Score: Brain, Mind, and Body in the Healing of Trauma* (Penguin Books, 2015).

Korean Recovery Recipes

1. "Asian Pear vs. Bosc Pear: What Is the Difference?" Versus (n.d.). https:// versus.com/en/asian-pear-vs-bosc-pear.

2. Young Hyun Hwang and J. C. Lee, "Variation of Asparagine and Aspartic Acid Contents in Soybean Sprouts," *KoreaScience*, Korean Society of Crop Science (Korea Republic) (1996).

3. Dhan Prakash et al., "Antioxidant and Free Radical-Scavenging Activities of Seeds and Agri-Wastes of Some Varieties of Soybean (*Glycine max*)," *Food Chemistry* 104, no. 2 (2007), 783–90. https://doi.org/10.1016/j .foodchem.2006.12.029.

4. "내손안에 동의보감," n.d. https://kc.mediclassics.kr/cont/contents.do? mobile_content_seq=30192#contentsListScroll_30192.

5. Ming-Yue Ji et al., "The Pharmacological Effects and Health Benefits of *Platycodon grandiflorus*—A Medicine Food Homology Species," *Foods* 9(2), 142 (2020). https://doi.org /10.3390 /foods9020142.

Listen to Your Body

1. "Chronic Daily Headaches," Mayo Clinic, accessed April 9, 2019. https:// www.mayoclinic.org/diseases-conditions/chronic-daily-headaches/ symptoms-causes/syc-20370891.

2. Jesús Peteiro et al., "Prediction of Cardiovascular, Cancer and Non-cardiovascular Non-cancer Death by Exercise Echocardiography," *European Journal of Preventive Cardiology*, 27(19) (2020), 2151–54. https://doi.org/10.1177/2047487319869692.

3. "내 손안에 동의보감," n.d. https://kc.mediclassics.kr/cont/contents.do?-mobile_content_seq=30192#contentsListScroll_30192.

Jeong: The Invisible Embrace

1. Christopher K. Chung and Samson J. Cho, "Conceptualization of Jeong and Dynamics of Hwabyung," *Psychiatry Investigation* 3, no. 1 (2006): 46–54.

2. Robert Waldinger and Marc Schulz, *The Good Life: Lessons from the World's Longest Scientific Study of Happiness* (Simon & Schuster, 2023).

3. Liz Mineo, "Harvard Study, Almost 80 Years Old, Has Proved that Embracing Community Helps Us Live Longer, and Be Happier," *Harvard Gazette*, April 11, 2017. https://news.harvard.edu/gazette/story/2017/04/over-nearly-80-years-harvard-study-has-been-showing-how-to-live-a-healthy-and-happy-life/.

4. Social Isolation and Loneliness in Older Adults. National Academies Press eBooks, 2020. https://doi.org/10.17226/25663.

Recipes

Index

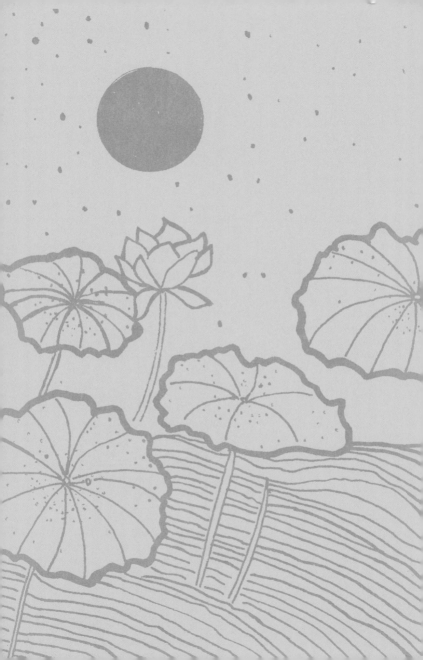